Nematology - Concepts, Diagnosis and Control
http://dx.doi.org/10.5772/66851
Edited by Mohammad Manjur Shah and Mohammad Mahamood

Contributors

Hugues Baimey, Charles Mackenzie, Ashley Braman, Roger Hauptman, Timothy Geary, Mohammad Manjur Shah, Mohammad Mahamood, Dimitris Tsaltas, Michalakis Christoforou, Michael Orford, Fábia Lima, Valdir Correa, Seloame Tatu Nyaku, Antoine Affokpon, Agyemang Danquah, Collison Brentu, Muying Ying, Gregory Bernard

Published by InTech
Janeza Trdine 9, 51000 Rijeka, Croatia

Publishing Process Manager Maja Bozicevic
Technical Editor SPi Global
Cover InTech Design team

First published August, 2017
Printed in Croatia
Legal deposit, Croatia: National and University Library in Zagreb

Additional hard copies can be obtained from orders@intechopen.com

Nematology - Concepts, Diagnosis and Control, Edited by Mohammad Manjur Shah and Mohammad Mahamood
p. cm.
Print ISBN 978-953-51-3415-2
Online ISBN 978-953-51-3416-9

For EU product safety concerns:
IN TECH d.o.o., Prolaz Marije Krucifikse Kozulić 3, 51000 Rijeka, Croatia,
info@intechopen.com or visit our website at intechopen.com.

Meet the editors

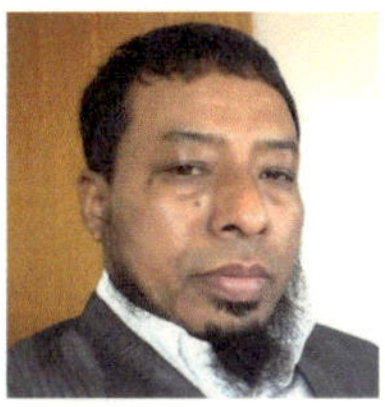

Dr. Mohammad Manjur Shah obtained his PhD degree from Aligarh Muslim University in the year 2003. He has been actively working on insect parasitic nematodes since 1998, and he is the pioneer in the field from the entire Northeast part of India. He has presented his findings in several conferences and published his articles in reputed international journals like Acta Parasitologica, Biologia, Zootaxa, Journal of Biology and Nature, Journal of Parasitic Diseases, Parassitologia, etc. He completed his postdoctoral fellowship twice under Ministry of Science and Technology, Government of India, before joining as Senior Asst. Professor at Northwest University, Kano, Nigeria. Apart from the present book, he edited two books with InTechOpen. He is also a reviewer of several journals of international repute.

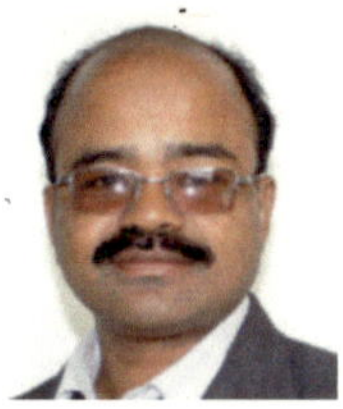

Dr. Mohammad Mahamood (MSc, MPhil, and PhD in Nematology-Zoology, Aligarh Muslim University) is an Assistant Professor in the School of Life and Allied Health Sciences, Glocal University, Saharanpur, UP, India. He has been a recipient of several prestigious scholarships. His experience in the fields of nematode biodiversity and ecology spans nearly two decades. He has previously served in the Department of Zoology, AMU, India and the Chinese Academy of Sciences, Shenyang, China, as a faculty member. Almost all the works of Dr. Mahamood are published in the journals of international repute including that of Nature Publishing House. His latest book, *Soil Nematodes of Grasslands in Northern China*, is published in Academic Press, Elsevier Publications.

Contents

Preface

Nematodes are a group of lesser-known but the most abundant group of multicellular organisms on earth. Nematology being an established discipline covers a wide range of area ranging from basic aspect (study of life cycle, ecology, epidemiology, taxonomy, biodiversity, biocontrol, etc.) to the advanced and applied aspects involving recent advances in molecular techniques that greatly enhanced our understanding right from the stage of proper identification of the organism under study that ultimately leads to diagnosis, treatment in the case of animal parasitic nematodes, and finally devising control strategies.

The book is mainly intended for biologists in general and nematologists in particular. The book was edited by collecting expert opinion of the scientific community in the field of nematology from various countries. The entire book contains up-to-date information having eight chapters spread over two sections; the first section deals with recent nematode diagnostic methods and tools, while the second section deals with control of nematodes. The book is well illustrated. Recent advances in basic and applied approaches including research on genetics of nematodes will assist in developing an opportunity to contribute at many different levels of research, including the development of new diagnostic tools and their control strategies.

This book discusses the following topics: the role of nematodes in our life (in agriculture, ecosystem functioning, experimental biology, ecological studies, pest management programs, or biocontrol), identification of GRSPs in nematode genomes, novel way for the diagnosis of pathogenic nematodes involving various recent molecular techniques, other methodologies for successful control of termites, evolution of plant-parasitic nematodes, viability of adult filarial nematode parasites, the impact of plant-parasitic nematodes on crops, and harnessing useful rhizosphere microorganisms for nematode control. The book also encompasses on classical study, molecular study, bioinformatics in nematology, biodiversity analysis, and culturing of nematodes in laboratory condition. I hope this book will surely find its wider application for current as well as future researchers as an easy reference book.

I am very much thankful to the Publishing Process Manager Ms. Maja Bozicevic for giving me cooperation throughout the process; without her initiative and help, this book would never have come to light. I also wish to thank all the technical staff associated with publication of the book (both online and in print edition).

Dr. Mohammad Manjur Shah
Sr. Asst. Professor
Dept. of Biological Sciences
Northwest University, Kano, Nigeria

Dr. Mohammad Mahamood
Asst. Professor
Glocal University, UP, India

Section 1

Recent Nematode Diagnostic Methods and Tools

Chapter 1

Introductory Chapter: Nematodes - A Lesser Known Group of Organisms

Mohammad Manjur Shah and
Mohammad Mahamood

Additional information is available at the end of the chapter

http://dx.doi.org/10.5772/intechopen.68589

1. Introduction

Nematodes are a group of lesser-known but the most abundant group of multicellular organisms on earth. They can be defined as a group of thread/worm-like, transparent, bilaterally symmetrical, pseudocoelomate and multicellular organisms that are free-living or parasitic to plants or animals. Numerically, they form the most abundant phylum within the meio- and mesofauna. However, for many of us, nematodes are something unseen and unheard. It is assumed to be due to their small size as well as their habit of remaining hidden in soil, water, plant and animal tissues. Nematodes, being ubiquitous, are associated with plants, insects, other invertebrate and vertebrate animals including domestic animals and even human beings. They exhibit different modes of life—parasitic (plant and animal), free-living, predatory, insect associates, entomopathogenic, terrestrial, aquatic (marine and freshwater) etc. The plant parasites may be migratory ectoparasites (feeding at different places but the body remaining outside of plant tissue) or migratory endoparasites (feeding at different places at the same time migrates inside the plant tissue) and some of them may be sedentary (in the forms with obese females like *Meloidogyne* sp.). Some are semiendoparasites (half of the body embedded in plant tissues while half remains outside), for example, *Tylenchulus semipenetrans*.

2. Brief history

Our knowledge of animal parasitic nematodes is much more ancient than that of plant-parasitic and free-living forms. Animal parasitic forms were known to us as early as 1500 BC. Large round worm like *Ascaris lumbricoides* and the dreaded Guinea worm, *Dracunculus medinensis*, etc., were known at that time [1]. On the other hand, soil nematodes remained unknown to us for a long period of time. It is assumed that this is due to the hidden mode of life these organisms lead as well as due to their minute size. Borellus [2] was the first to observe a free-living nematode, *Turbatrix aceti* (vinegar eel). Needham [3] reported the first plant-parasitic nematode. Systematics of nematodes was first published by Rudolphi [4]. Leidy [5] was the first one to describe a freshwater nematode, *Tobriluslongus*. Dujardin [6] for the first time described a dorylaim nematode, *Dorylaimus stagnalis*.

It is almost impossible to make a list of all nematologists the world has had so far. However, an effort is being made to highlight some of the important contributions made by the past and present nematologists. In nematode taxonomy, Bastian [7] made a historic contribution through his descriptions of 100 new species under 23 new and 7 known genera. Schneider [8] and Bütschli [9, 10] gave detailed accounts of free-living nematodes. Örley [11] provided the first comprehensive survey on the taxonomy of free-living nematodes which included 202 species belonging to 27 genera. Modern generic and specific descriptions are based mainly on the de Man's works [12]. His monograph [13] is regarded the "Bible of Nematologists" and his indices for expressing nematode morphometric values are still used with some modifications and additions. Cobb is considered as the "Father of Nematology in the United States." He published a series of very valuable papers.

There are several other nematologists whose contributions deserve to be mentioned. Filipjev [14–16] made significant changes in the classification of nematodes. Micoletzky [17] reported 142 genera and 931 species. The present classification of Nematoda is mainly based on the hypothesis of Paramonov & Filipjev. Chitwood's book [18] "An Introduction to Nematology" is a golden piece of work in the history of Nematology. Valuable contributions made by Thorne in the form of his monographs on Dorylaims [19], Cephalobidae [20] and Tylenchida [21], and in the form of his book [22] "Principles of Nematology" need special mention. Goodey [23] gave much information related to soil and freshwater nematodes. Contributions made by Meyl [24], Grasse [25]and Gerlach & Riemann [26, 27] still prove to be milestones in terms of changes in nomenclature, synonymisations and reviews. Andrássy's contributions in the field of nematode taxonomy [28–32] will always remain a great asset of Nematology forever. Blaxter et al. [33] and De Ley & Blaxter [34] revised the classification of phylum Nematoda based on molecular and morphological characters. Eyualem et al. [35], Steiner [35, 36–43], Füchs [44–48], Rahm [49–52], Allgen [53–56], Altherr [57–60], Pearse [61], Hirschmann [11, 62, 63], Kirjanova [64–66], Wieser [67–69], Timm [70], Golden [71], Loof [72–74], Coomans et al. [75], Inglis [76], etc., also contributed significantly to the field of Nematology. Contributions made by Siddiqi [77], Jairajpuri and Ahmad [78] are highly valued.

3. Smart lifestyle of smart organisms

It is impossible to think of a habitat, macro or micro, without nematodes like hot springs, low oxygen conditions, acid environments, rocky mountains, deep sea trenches, polar regions, aerial region, subterranean region, decaying organic debris, plant roots, stems, flowers and seeds. Thus, in habitat diversity, nematodes are the masters. This vast distribution may be attributed to their surprisingly versatile life. Nematodes may be bacterial and fungal feeders, parasites of plant, predators and parasites of animals (insects to humans and livestock). Many species cause deaths to insects (entomopathogenic). Such nematodes that kill economically important pests are popularly called as "Farmers best friend" [79]. Some nematodes may simply develop phoretic relationship (meant for only transport from one place to other) with the insects.

Nematode body is described by many as "tube within a tube." Nematodes have a very simple body plan. However, they can successfully survive a wide range of geo-physico-chemical conditions. In unfavorable conditions, they can switch their food preference, a condition known as omnivory. They can survive without any detectable metabolic activity (*cryptobiosis*) or simply they can lower their rate of metabolism (*dormancy*). The young ones (juveniles) can also survive unfavorable conditions through a kind of survival stage in which metabolic activities are suppressed (*dauer stages*). Some species can survive complete dryness.

So far, Arthropoda is the largest phylum in the kingdom Animalia. However, nematodes are the most abundant organisms. Four of every five multicellular animals on our planet are nematodes [79]. Nearly 90% of the multicellular animals on earth are nematodes [12, 80, 81]. An average of 15,000–20,000 juveniles of *Anguina tritici* is present in a single wheat gall. Many million individuals per m^2 in soil and bottom sediments of aquatic habitats may be present and it is not uncommon to find more than 50 species in a handful of soil. Nathan Augustus Cobb, referred to as the Father of Nematology in the United States [13] very rightly said, "*If all the matter in the universe except nematodes were swept away, our world would still be recognizable, and if, as disembodied spirits, we could then investigate it, we should find its mountains, hills, vales, rivers, lakes, and oceans represented by a film of nematodes.*"

4. Role of nematodes in our life

In agriculture: Most of the soil nematodes are microscopic. However, their direct and indirect roles in a country's economy are massive. Annual crop losses due to nematodes have been estimated to more or less $80 billion. In many developing countries, the population increases at a very fast pace while the size of fertile land decreases due to industrialization, expansion of urban area, transport system, etc.

In ecosystem functioning: In the food chain of subterranean ecosystem, nematodes play a very important role. Many of them are bacterial and fungal feeders which contribute to decomposition of organic materials and thus increase fertility, while many others are parasites of plants attacking a wide range of plants. Many others attack human beings and livestock. A good number of them are predators and thus feed on soil microarthropods, nematodes, etc.

In experimental biology: A good number of them have successfully been used as experimental models, for example, *Caenorhabditis elegans* and *Pristionchus pacificus*. Nematodes, specially the bacterial and fungal feeders, are easy to culture in the laboratory. They can complete the whole life cycle in a few days. Many trials can be done on several generations in a short period of time. As their body is transparent, their internal structures can be observed without going through the process of tedious dissections.

In ecological studies: All of the species are equally good for ecological studies. There are several other species which are considered to be reliable bioindicators too. Nematode community structure can be used as a bioindicator in environmental monitoring [52].

In pest management programs: The entomopathogenic nematodes like the species of *Steinernema, Heterorhabditis, Neosteinernema*, etc., have been used in successful management of many economically important insect pests [82].

5. External and internal morphology of nematodes

With a few exceptions, all the nematodes are vermiform (worm-like). They show a great range of species-specific variability in their body morphologies.

Body shape or body posture: Generally, nematodes have elongated, spindle-shaped body. However, pear-shaped, lemon-shaped or saccate body also occurs. Nematode body usually tapers toward anterior (head) and posterior ends. Nematodes' body posture on head is interestingly very specific. The body may remain straight or slightly/strongly curved ventrally; or spiraled or exceptionally dorsally curved.

Body size: Nematodes show a great range of variability in their body size. It ranges from less than 82 μm (*Grifiella minutum*—marine) to more than 8 meter (*Placentonema gigantissima*—placenta of whale). Most of the free-living and plant-parasitic nematodes are small in size, while the predatory nematodes are large.

Body wall: The outer body wall (exoskeleton) of nematode is known as cuticle. Externally, it bears longitudinal or transverse striations or both. Besides the longitudinal and transverse striations, the cuticle may possess differently modified structures called cuticular ornamentations—dots, warts, depressions, elevations, projections or spines from the posterior margins of the annules. Below the cuticle, there lies the hypodermis and the musculature. The cuticle is made of mainly protein with small amounts of lipids and carbohydrates. It is semipermeable. Cuticle varies from species to species in terms of thickness and structure. It is mainly composed of three layers—cortical layer, median layer and basal layer. The number of layers in the cuticle is more in animal parasitic forms (e.g., 7–9 layers in *Ascaris*).

Hypodermis: As has been mentioned above, the hypodermis lies below the cuticle. It is a thin layer and is characterized by the presence of four longitudinal invaginations also called chords (dorsal—1, ventral—1 and laterals—2) in the coelomic cavity.

Somatic musculature: It is a layer of spindle-shaped muscle cells attached to the hypodermis. Each of these muscle cells has sarcoplasmic and fibrillar parts.

Lip or cephalic region: Lip region is the anteriormost part of the body and it differs in different groups of nematodes. It may be continuous or set off from the body.

Lips and labial papillae: There are six lips arranged circularly around the oral opening. Two of them are in the lateral sectors, two are in subventral sectors and two are in subdorsal sectors. Each lip carries three papillae except the laterals which carry two papillae. The labial papillae are arranged in inner and outer circlets. There is only one papilla on each lip in the inner circlet, while two papillae each are there on each lip in the submedian sectors. The lateral lips carry one papilla each.

Cephalic framework: It is a ring or basket-like cuticularized structure present around the stoma. It may be weakly or strongly cuticularized and it varies from species to species.

Amphid: It is a paired structure considered to be chemoreceptor organs. These are present in the lateral sectors of the body in the anterior esophageal region. The amphids open to exterior and the openings of amphids may be circular, oval, slit-like or pore-like and may be located on the lateral lips or close to or far posterior to them.

Deirids: Like amphids, deirids are also paired structures. They are circular, thickened and are present on cuticle in the mid-lateral sectors in the pharyngeal region around the level of excretory pore.

Phasmids: Phasmids are also circular and paired and are present in the mid-lateral regions. Generally, these are present posterior to anus (females) or cloaca (males). However, their positions may be adanal, pre-anal or even further anterior. Either the phasmids may be just opposite to each other or one of these may be shifted anterior or posterior.

Stoma: The anteriormost part of the digestive tract is the stoma. It varies in shape and size in different nematode groups having different food and feeding habits. Bacterial and fungal feeders have tubular or funnel-shaped or barrel-shaped stoma (**Figure 1(A), (B)**), whereas plant-parasitic tylenchids (**Figure 1(C)**) and aphelenchids have a protractible, hypodermic needle-like stylet/spear. The predators, on the other hand, have wide and spacious stoma which may or may not be provided with tooth, teeth or denticles (**Figure 1(E)** and **(F)**). The terminology used for the feeding apparatus is different in different nematode groups. In the dorylaim nematodes, it is called odontostyle, while in nygolaims, it is named onchiostyle. In case of mononchs, it is simply called buccal/stomal cavity. The buccal cavity in mononchs is generally provided with dorsal tooth, a pair of subventral teeth, denticles, etc.

Esophagus: It is also called pharynx. It is a roughly tubular structure. It connects the stoma with intestine. It varies in shape and size in different groups. In Tylenchida and Rhabditida, it is tripartite (having three different parts) (**Figures 2(A)**, **(B)** and **3**).

Esophageal glands: These are also called as pharyngeal or salivary glands. Esophageal glands are nothing but unicellular, uninucleate cells found embedded in pharyngeal tissue. There is variation in the number of these glands in different groups. Tylenchids usually have three glands, while the dorylaims have five glands. In tylenchs, the glands may extend over the intestine forming a kind of lobe.

Esophago-intestinal junction: It is also called cardia. It is a disc or tongue-like structure. It connects the pharynx with intestine. It prevents the food in intestine from coming back to pharynx.

Intestine: It is a tubular structure made up of a single layer of comparatively large cells. It is the longest part in the digestive system connecting the cardia anteriorly and the rectum (in all groups except dorylaims) or prerectum posteriorly (dorylaims).

Prerectum: In Dorylaimida, the intestine posteriorly connects with prerectum. It is different from the intestine proper in color, thickness, texture of the food containing in it. The length of prerectum is variable and is different from species to species.

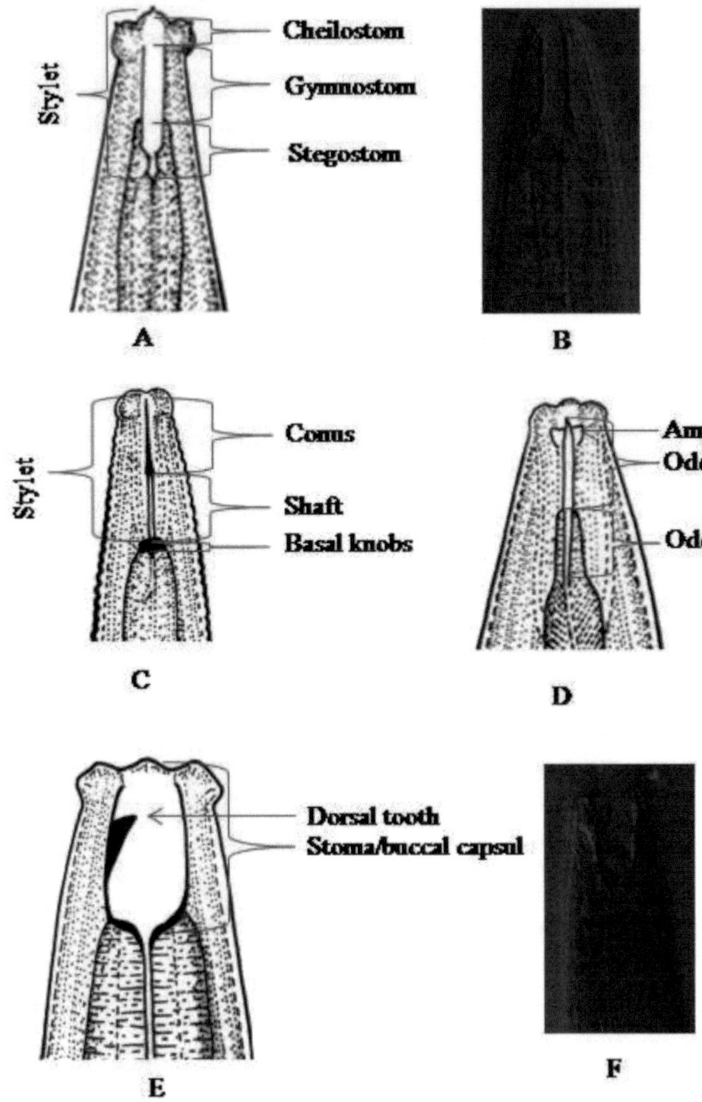

Figure 1. (A) Rhabditid (bacterial & fungal feeder) stoma, (B) photograph of rhabditid stoma, (C) Tylenchida (plant-parasitic) stoma, (D) Dorylaim (predatory, some are plant parasites) stoma, (E) Mononchid (predator) stoma, (F) photograph of Mononchid stoma.

Rectum: It connects anteriorly with intestine or prerectum and posteriorly with anus. The junction with intestine is provided with sphincter (circular-contractile ring made of muscles) muscles. In many species, the anterior end of rectum may carry three unicellular glands.

Anus/cloaca: Females have separate openings for both digestive and reproductive systems—anus and vulva. Anus is the end point of the rectum. It opens to the exterior. Males, on the other hand, have a common opening for both digestive and reproductive systems to the exterior and is called cloaca.

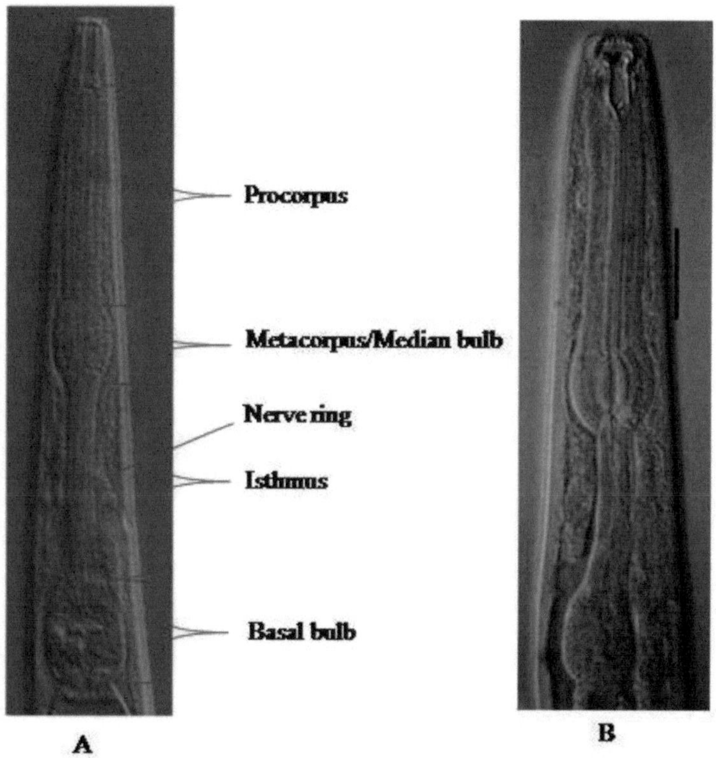

Figure 2. (A) Rhabditid (bacterivorous) pharynx, (B) Diplogastrid (omnivore-predator) pharnyx.

Female reproductive system: Reproductive system in females is composed of ovary, oviduct, spermatheca, uterus, vagina and vulva. The reproductive system may be single (*monodelphic*) or paired (*didelphic*). The gonad(s) may be positioned anterior to vulva (*prodelphic*) or posterior to the vulva (*opisthodelphic*), or on both the sides (*amphidelphic*). Both the reproductive systems may be positioned on the same side (*didelphic-prodelphic*, e.g., *Meloidogyne*). A nonfunctional gonad which is also reduced in size may be present in addition to the functional one. This condition is known *pseudo-prodelphic* (anterior) or *pseudo-opisthodelphic* (posterior) gonad. The reduced, nonfunctional branch is called as *prevulval uterine sac* (anterior) or *postvulval uterine sac* (posterior).

Male reproductive system: The components of male reproductive system are very important for proper identification. In many instances, studying only the female characteristics is not enough for species level identification. The male sexual characters comprise of testis, seminal vesicle, ejaculatory duct, cloacal chamber and its associated glands, spicules, gubernaculum, lateral guiding pieces, copulatory muscles, genital papillae and bursa. Testis may be single (*monorchic*) or paired (*diorchic*). The testis is outstretched with the tip directed anteriorly in monorchic condition. However, in diorchic condition, one testis is placed in reversed condition with the whole of it directing the opposite side.

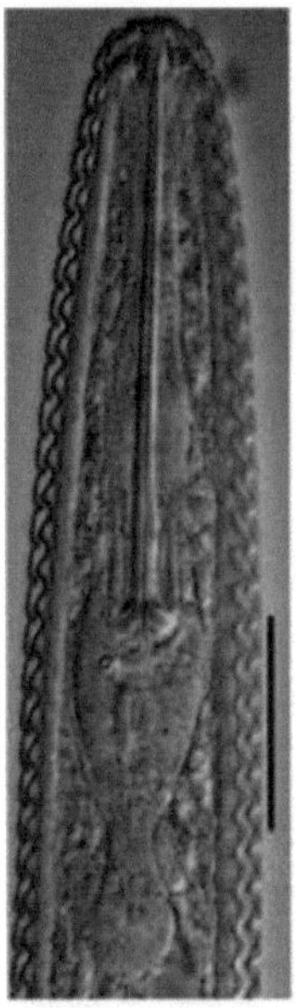

Figure 3. Criconematid (plant-parasitic) pharnyx (procorpus and metacorpus fused, isthmus very short, basal bulb recorded.

Tail: Tail in nematodes may be of different shapes and lengths. It may be short, long, long conoid, whip-like, filamentous, conoid, digitate, clavate, hemispheroid, etc. It may be with phasmids, scutella (singular—scutellum), caudal glands, caudal pores, caudal setae, spinneret, mucro, etc. Tail may differ in shape and length in different sexes.

6. Collection and processing of samples

Soil samples: The soil samples should be taken from a depth of 10–25 cm after removing the topmost dry layer of soil and should be kept in airtight polythene bags. Each sample should be tied so that the soil particles are not disturbed. Loosely tied soil samples may not give a good collection of nematodes as they may die due to desiccation before processing the samples. All relevant information such as host, locality, and date of collection should also be noted. Till further processing the samples should be kept undisturbed, away from sunlight at 20–25°C.

Plant materials: For studying nematodes which are ectoparasites of roots, the samples should be collected from around the roots of the host plant. Effort should be made to collect the fine roots too. For endoparasitic nematodes, direct observation of the affected parts after staining is suitable.

Staining the roots with acid fuchsin solution: First, prepare stock solution of acid fuchsin by dissolving 3.5 g of acid fuchsin in 250 ml acetic acid and then increase the volume up to 1000 ml by adding distilled water. Secondly, dip the roots thoroughly in 5.25% NaOCl and keep for about 4 min. Thirdly, wash the roots by using tap water for about 45 s and then keep the roots immersed in water for 15 min to avoid any residue of NaOCl. It may otherwise affect staining. Now, the roots should be transferred to a glass beaker containing 30–50 ml of tap water. Take 1 ml of stock solution and pour into the glass beaker containing roots and tap water. Boil the same for about 30 s. Let it cool down to room temperature and drain the stained solution. Rinse the roots again in running tap water. Now, the roots can be teased with the help of needles under a stereoscopic microscope to examine the presence of any endo- or semiendoparasitic nematodes such as *Meloidogyne incognita, Tylenchulus semipenetrans*, etc.

Isolation of nematodes from soil samples: There are many techniques employed to isolate nematodes from soil samples. Some of them are Oostenbrink's elutriator, Seinhort's elutriator, Cobb's decanting and sieving technique, Baermann's funnel technique, Maceration-filtration technique, Mistifier extraction technique, Sugar floatation technique, etc. However, a combination of Cobb's [83] decanting and sieving technique and Baermann's funnel technique is commonly used in a slightly modified way. It is very good to isolate vermiform, active nematodes. The drawback of this technique is that it cannot isolate the immobile, inactive individuals and also the eggs.

Modified Cobb's decanting and sieving technique: In this, around 500 cc of sample is taken in a bucket and mixed with water thoroughly. The debris and pebbles, if present, are removed, and soil crumbs (in case of soil samples) are broken manually. The bucket is then filled with water and the suspension is stirred thoroughly to make it homogeneous. It is then left undisturbed for about half a minute so as to allow the heavy soil particles to settle down to the bottom of the bucket. The suspension is then passed into another bucket through a coarse sieve (2 mm pore size), which retains debris, roots and leaves. The suspension in the second bucket is again stirred thoroughly and left for another half a minute and then poured through a BSS 300mesh sieve (pore size 53 μm). The catch on the sieve containing nematodes and very fine soil particles is collected in a beaker. The process is repeated twice for good recovery of nematodes.

Modified Baermann's funnel technique: The residue collected in the beaker is poured on a small coarse sieve which is already lined with tissue paper. The small coarse sieve is then placed in a Baermann's funnel fitted with stoppered rubber tubing. Tap water is slowly poured into the funnel until it touched the bottom of the sieve. Care should be taken to avoid trapping of air bubbles at the bottom of the sieve as the nematodes containing in the coarse sieve will not migrate down the funnel in the area where there are bubbles. The nematodes will migrate from the sieve into the clear water of the funnel and settle at bottom. After 24 h, a small amount of water containing the nematodes can be drained from the funnel into a glass cavity block.

Killing and fixation: The nematodes collected in cavity blocks should be left undisturbed for some time so as to allow them to settle to the bottom of the cavity blocks. Excess water should then be removed with a fine dropper. Disposable syringe with very fine hypodermic needle can be easier to handle for removing excess water from the cavity blocks. Use of a hot fixative will simultaneously kill and fix the nematodes. There are several fixatives like TAF (8 ml formalin + 2 ml triethanolamine + 90 ml distilled water), FG (8 ml formalin + 2 ml glycerin + 90 ml distilled water).

Dehydration: After 24 h of fixation, the nematodes should be transferred into a mixture of glycerin-alcohol (5 parts glycerin + 95 parts 30% alcohol) in a small cavity block. Picking individually and transferring several nematodes is not easy, and it is not good for health too as the fixative is formaldehyde-based. It can be avoided by simply drawing the fixative out of the cavity block by using a fine-tipped dropper or a disposable syringe. Then, remove the fixative as much as possible and add glycerin-alcohol and keep the same in desiccator containing anhydrous fused calcium chloride. In 3–4 weeks' time, the nematodes will be dehydrated completely.

Mounting and sealing: Take a clean glass slide and place a small drop of anhydrous glycerin and transfer the nematodes from the cavity block to this drop and make them settle on the surface of the slide. Take 3 cubes of wax (approximately 2 mm^2) and place around the glycerin drop at around 120° to each other. It is preferable to place three pieces of glass wool of same thickness as of the nematodes around the nematodes to prevent flattening. Take a circular glass cover slip (18 mm diameter) and gently place on it and keep the slide on a hot plate to allow the wax to melt and seal the slide.

Measurements and drawing: For taxonomic studies or for any pest-management program, proper identification is the key to success. For proper identification, measurements of different body parts are inevitable. All measurements can be made on specimens mounted in dehydrated glycerine with an ocular micrometer. The ocular micrometer should be calibrated first by using a stage micrometer. For denoting dimensions of nematode, De Man [84] introduced a system. It was further modified in 1880. There have been many changes made by some famous nematologists like Cobb [26], Thorne [20], Caveness [85], etc. Besides those changes, these morphometric parameters are still known as the De Man's indices/formula and are given below.

n = Number of specimens measured.

L = Body length.

V = Distance from anterior end to vulva/total body length ×100.

a = Body length/greatest body diameter.

b = Body length/length of pharynx.

b′ = Body length/distance of base esophageal glands from anterior end.

c = Body length/tail length.

c′ = Tail length/diameter of tail at anus or cloaca.

s = Stylet length/diameter of body at base of stylet.

T = % Total length of testis relative to total body length.

G^1 = % Total length of anterior female gonad in relation to total body length.

G_2 = % Total length of posterior female gonad in relation to total body length.

7. Nematode trophic groups

Ecological studies using nematodes as models use the feeding habit as the basis of categorization. Nematodes show all possible modes of feeding. Such type of classification is far away from the systematics of the nematode species concerned. All the species sharing a common mode of feeding are considered in a single category. Many nematode ecologists have proposed several trophic groups. The trophic groups of nematodes are herein proposed as follows -

1. *Plant-feeding*: This group includes those nematodes feeding on plant tissues. Such nematodes possess a spear (Tylenchida) or an odontostyle (Dorylaimida). This group may be further divided into

   i) Migratory ectoparasites—This group is represented by those species which feed at different places but never enter into the plant tissue. They can penetrate the stylet deep into the cortex, for example, members of the family Dolichodoridae, Criconematidae, etc. The feeding may also be restricted only to the epidermal cells and root hairs as in case of the members of the families Tylenchidae, Psilenchidae, etc., in which the stylet is not so strong.

   ii) Migratory endoparasites—It is represented by those nematodes which migrate inside plant tissues, for example, *Radopholus*.

   iii) Sedentary endoparasites—It includes the groups in which the females become obese, for example, *Meloidogyne*.

   iv) Semiendoparasites—This group includes those nematodes in which half of the body is embedded inside plant tissues, while the rest of the body is exposed to the external environment, for example *Tylenchulus*.

2. *Bacterial-feeding*: This group is represented by those nematodes having cylindrical or barrel-shaped or slightly wide feeding apparatus such as rhabditid and diplogastrid species.

3. *Omnivore-predators*: This type of feeding habit is found in some diplogastrid species in which the stoma is provided with armatures such as tooth, teeth, denticles, etc.

4. *Predatory*: Many nematode species of Mononchida, Dorylaimida (Naigolaimina), Rhabditida (Diplogastrina) live on the soil microarthropods, nematodes, etc.

Author details

Mohammad Manjur Shah[1]* and Mohammad Mahamood[2]

*Address all correspondence to: mmanjurshah@gmail.com

1 Department of Biological Science, Northwest University, Kano, Nigeria

2 School of Life and Allied Health Sciences, Glocal University, Saharanpur, India

References

[1] Hoeppli R. Parasites and parasitic infections in early science and medicine. Singapore, Singapore: University of Malaya Press: 1959

[2] Borellus P. 'Observatiouum Micioscopicarum Cenluria,' Hagoe coniil.is.384, Paris. 1656

[3] Needham F. An account of some new microscopical discoveries. London. 1743. p. 126

[4] Rudolphi CA. Entozoorum synopsis cui acceduntmantesia duplex et indices locupletissimi. Berolini, Sumtibus A. Rücker 1819. pp. 811

[5] Leidy J. Contributions to helminthology. Proceedings of the Academy of Natural Sciences of Philadelphia. 1851;**5**:205-209, 224-227

[6] Dujardin F. Histoire naturelle des helminthes ouversintestinaux. De L'imprimerie de Crapelet, Rue de Vaugirard Paris. 1845. pp. 654

[7] Bastian HC. Monograph on the Anguillulidae, or free Nematoids, marine, land and freshwater; With descriptions of 100 new species. Transactions of the Linnaean Society of London. 1865;**25**:73-184

[8] Schneider AF. Monographie der Nematoden. Georg Reimer, Berlin. 1866. pp. 357.

[9] Bütschli O. Beiträgezur Kenntnis der freilebenden Nematoden. Nov Acta der Kaiserlich-Leopoldinsch-carolinischen Deutschen Akademie der Naturforscher. 1873;**36**:3-144

[10] Bütschli O. Untersuchungenüberfreilebende Nematoden und die Gattung Chaetonotus. Zeitschriftfürwissenchaftliche Zoologie. 1876;**26**:363-413

[11] Kirjanova ES. Nematodypoehvykholkovogopolja i theliny v Golodnoj step (Uzbekistan). (In Russian). Trudy Zoologicheskogo Instituta Akademiya Nauk SSSR. 1951;**9**:625-657

[12] De Man JG. Onderzoekingen over vrij in de aardelevende Nematoden. Tijdachr. Nederl. Kierk. Ver. 1876;**2**:78-196

[13] De Man JG. Die frei in der reinen Erde und imsüssen Wasserlebenden Nematoden der niederländischen Fauna. Einesystematisch-faunistische Monographie, E. J. Brill, Leiden. 1884;1-206

[14] Filipjev I. Free-living marine nematodes of the Sevastopol area. Trudy Osoboi Zoologicheskoi laboratorii i Sebastopol'skoibiologicheskoistantsii. 1918;**4**:1-350

[15] Filipjev I. Free-living marine nematodes of the Sevastopol area. Trudy Osoboi Zoologicheskoilaboratorii i Sebastopol'skoibiologicheskoistantsii. 1921;**4**:351-614

[16] Filipjev I. The classification of the free-living nematodes and their relation to the parasitic nematodes. Smithsonian Miscellaneous Collections (Washington). 1934;**89**:1-63

[17] Micoletzky H. Die freilebenden Erd-Nematoden mitbesonderer Berücksichtigung der steiermark und der Bukowina, Zugleichmiteiner revision sämtlichernichtmariner, freilebender Nematoden in Form von Genus-Beschreibungen und Bestimmungsschlüsse. Archivfür Naturgeschichte Abteilung. 1922;**87**:1-650

[18] Chitwood BG, Chitwood MB. Introduction to Nematology. Baltimore: Monumental Printing Company; revised edition. 1950. p. 213

[19] Thorne G. A revision of the nematode family Cephalobidae Chitwood and Chitwood, 1934. Proceedings of the Helminthological Society of Washington. 1937;**4**:1-16

[20] Thorne G. On the classification of the Tylenchida, new order (Nematoda, Phasmidia). Proceedings of Helminthological Society Washington. 1949;**16**:37-73

[21] Thorne G. Principles of Nematology. New York: McGraw-Hill Company, Inc; 1961. p. 553

[22] Goodey T. Soil and Fresh Water Nematodes – A Monograph. Methuen & Co. Ltd. London. 1951. pp. 390

[23] Meyl AH. Die freilebendenErd- und Süßwassernematoden (Fadenwürmer). In: Die TierweltMitteleuropas. Brohmer P, Ehrmann P, Ulmer G, editors. 1960/1961;**1**:1-164

[24] Grasse PP. Traité de Zoologie, Tome IV, Fascicule 2-3, Masson, Paris. 1965

[25] Gerlach SA, Riemann F. The Bremerhaven checklist of aquatic nematodes. Veröffentlichungen Institutfür Meeresforschung Bremerhaven, Supplement. 1973;**4**:1-404

[26] Gerlach SA, Riemann F. The Bremerhaven checklist of aquatic nematodes. Veröffentlichungen Institutfür Meeresforschung Bremerhaven, Supplement 1974;**4**:405-734

[27] Andrássy I. Evolution as a basis for the systematization of nematodes. Budapest. London, Pitman Publishing. 1976. pp. 288

[28] Andrássy I. Klasse Nematoda(Ordungen Monhysterida, Desmoscolecida, Araeolaimida, Chromadorida, Rhabditida). Stuttgart: Gustav Fischer Verlag; 1984; pp. 509

[29] Andrássy I. Free-living nematodes of Hungary (Nematodaerrantia). Czudi C, Mahunka S, editors. In: Paedozoologica Hungarica. 2005a; Vol. **I**, p. 518

[30] Andrássy I. Free-living nematodes of Hungary (Nematodaerrantia). Czudi C, Mahunka S, editors. In: Paedozoologica Hungarica. 2005b; Vol. **II**, p. 496

[31] Andrássy I. Free-living nematodes of Hungary (Nematodaerrantia). Czudi C, Mahunka S, editors. In: Paedozoologica Hungarica. 2005c; Vol. **III**, 608p

[32] Blaxter ML, De Ley P, Garey JR, Liu LX, Scheldeman P, Vierstraete A, Vanfleteren J R, Mackey LY, Dorris M, Frisse LM, Vida JT, Thomas WK. A molecular evolutionary framework for the phylum Nematoda. Nature. 1998;**392**:71-75

[33] De Ley P, Blaxter M. Systematic position and phylogeny. Lee DL, editor. In: The Biology of Nematodes. London, New York: Taylor and Francis; 2002. pp. 1-30

[34] Eyualem A, Traunspurger W, Andrássy I. Freshwater nematodes: Ecology and Taxonomy., Wallingford, Oxfordshire UK: CABI Publishing; 2006. p. 752

[35] Fuchs AG. Die Naturgeschichte der Nematoden und einigeranderererParasiten. 1. Des IpstypographusL.2. Des HylobiusabietisL. ZoologischeJahrbücher (Systematik). 1915;**38**:109-222

[36] Fuchs AG. NeueanBorken-und Rüsselkäfergebundene Nematoden, halbparasitische und Wohnungseinmieter. Zoologische Jahrbücher (Systematik). 1930;**59**:505-646

[37] Fuchs AG. Einigeneue Rhabditis-Arten. Zoologische Jahrbücher (Systematik). 1931;**62**: 119-148

[38] Füchs G. Neueparasitische und halbparasitische Nematodenbei Borkenkäfern und einigeandere Nematoden. 1. Teil. ZoologischeJahrbücher (Systematik). 1937;**70**:291-380

[39] Fuchs AG. Neueparasiten und halbparasitenbei Borkenkäfern und einigeandere Nematoden. Zoologische Jahrbücher (Systematik). 1938;**71**:123-190

[40] Steiner G. Procephalobusmycophilusn. g., n. sp. (Cephalobina), a nematode living in thesclerotia of the fungus Balansiaclaviceps. Proceedings of the Helminthological Society of Washington. 1934;**1**:56-58

[41] Steiner G. Opuscula miscellanea nematologica. III. Proceedings of the Helminthological Society of Washington. 1936a;**3**:16-22

[42] Golden AM. Taxonomy of the spiral nematodes (Rotylenchusand Helicotylenchus) and the developmental stages and host-parasite relationships of *R. buxophilusn.* sp., attacking boxwood. Maryland Agricultural Experimental Station Bulletin A. **85**. 1956;28

[43] Steiner G. Opuscula miscellanea nematologica VII. (I). Observations on nematodes associated with Irish potatoes grown in South Carolina. Proceedings of the Helminthological Society of Washington. 1938;**5**:35-40

[44] Steiner G. Freilebende Suisswasser nematoden ausperuanischen Hochgebirgsseen. Revue Suisse de Zoologie. 1920;**28**:11-44

[45] Steiner G. Parasitic nemas on peanuts in South Africa. Centralbl. Bakteriol. 1926;**67**:16-24

[46] Steiner G. Diplogasterentomophagan. sp., a new Diplogaster(Diplogastridae, Nematodes) found on a Pamphilusstellatus (CHRIST) (Tenthredinidae, Hymenoptera). Zoologischer Anzeiger.1929;**80**:143-145

[47] Steiner G. Some nemic parasites and associates of the mountain pine beetle (Dendroctonusmonticolae). Journal of agricultural Research. 1932;**45**:437-444

[48] Rahm G. BeitragzurKenntnis der Moostierwelt der preusischenRheinlande. I. Archiv fur Naturgeschichte 90 AS. 1924;174-176

[49] Rahm G. Alguns nematodes parasitas e semi-parasitas das plantascultureas do Brasil. Archivos do Instituto de Biológico de Defesa Agricola e Animal (Sao Paulo). 1928;**1**: 239-251

[50] Rahm G. Nematodes parasitas e semi-parasitas de diversasplantascultureas do Brasil. Archivos do Instituto de Biológico de defesa Agricola e Animal (Sao Paulo). 1929;**2**:67-136

[51] Huettel RN, Golden AM. Nathan Augustus Cobb: The Father of Nematology in the United States. Annual Review of Phytopathology. 1991;**29**:15-26

[52] Allgén C. Übereinigefreilebende Nematodenausdem Niederkongo. Zoologischer Anzeiger. 1933;**103**:312-320

[53] Allgén C. Die freilebenden Nematoden des Öresunds. Capita Zoologica. 1935;**6**: 5-192

[54] Allgén C. Weitere Untersuchuugenüberschwedische Nematoden. I. Glauxinemafilicaudatumn. gen.n.sp., eineneue Anguillulide von der Westküste Schwedens. Kungliga Fysiografiska Sällskapets Förhandlingar (Lund). 1947;**17**:73-78

[55] Allgén C. Übereinigefreilebende Süsswasser-Nematoden von Mt. Kenya (Brit. Ostafrika). Einkleiner Beitragzur Kenntnistropischer Nematoden. Ark FürZoologie. 1952;**2**: 139-157

[56] Altherr E. La faune des mines de Bex, aveeétudespéciale des Nématodes. Revue Suisse de Zoologie. 1938;**45**:567-720

[57] Altherr E. Les nématodes du Pare national suisse. (Nemaodeslibres du sol.).2e partie. Ergebnisse der Wissenschaftlichen Untersuchung des Schweizerischen. National Parks. 1952;**3**:315-356

[58] Altherr E. Contribution à la connaissance de la faunesablessubmergés en Lorraine. Nématodes. Annales de Spéléologie. 1963;**18**:53-98

[59] Altherr E. Nématodes des eauxstygorhitrales des Alpesautrichiennes. Revue Suisse de Zoologie. 1976;**83**:779-847

[60] Pearse AS. An introduction to Parasitology. Baltimore, USA: Thomas, C.C; 1942. p. 375

[61] Hirschmann H. Über das Vorkommenzweier Mundhöhlentypenbei Diplogasterlheritieri Maupas und Diplogasterbiformisn. sp. und dei Entstehungdieserhermaphordotischen Art ausDiplogasterlheritieri. I. Mitteilung. Zoologische Jahrbücher (Systematik). 1951;**80**: 132-170

[62] Hirschmann H. Die Nematoden der WassergrenzemittelfränkischerGewässer. Zoologische Jahrbücher (Systematik). 1952;**81**:313-364

[63] Hirschmann H. Comparative morphological studies on the soybean cyst nematode, Heteroderaglycinesand the clover cyst nematode, H. trifolii (Nematoda: Heteroderidae). Proceedings of Helminthological Society of Washington. 1956;**23**:140-151

[64] Kirjanova ES. Antarktic heskiepredstavitelipres novodnykh nematodroda Plectus Bastian (Nematodes, Plectidae).(In Russian). Information Bulletin of Soviet. Antarctic Expedition. 1958;**3**:101-103

[65] Kirjanova ES, Krall E. Paraziticheskienematodyrastenij i meryborby s nimi. Tom II. Leningrad. 1971. p. 523

[66] Wieser W. Die Beziehungzwischen Mundhöhlengestalt, Ernährungsweise und Vorkommenbeifreilebenden marinen Nematoden. Archiv Fur Zoologie. 1953;**4**:439-484

[67] Wieser W. Free-living marine nematodes. II. Chromadoroidea. ActaUniversitasis-Lundensis. 1954;**50**:1-148

[68] Wieser W. Free-living marine nematodes. III. Axonolaimoidea and Monhysteroidea. Report Lund University Chile Expedition. 1948-49. ActaUniversitatisLundensis(N.F.2). 1956;**52**:1-115

[69] Timm RW. Antarctic soil and freshwater nematodes from the McMurdo Sound Region. Proceedings of the Helminthological Society of Washington. 1971;**38**:42-52

[70] Steiner G. Opuscula miscellanea nematologica. IV. Proceedings of the Helminthological Society of Washington. 1936b;**3**:74-80

[71] Loof PAA. Free-living and plant-parasitic nematodes from Venezuela. Nematologica. 1964;**10**:201-300

[72] Loof PAA. Free-living and plant-parasitic nematodes from Spitzbergen, collected by Van Rossen, H. Mededelingen van de Landbouwhogeschool Wageningen. 1971;**71**:1-86

[73] Loof PAA. Freshwater nematodes from Suriname collected by J. Van der Land. Zoologische Verhandelingen. 1973;**129**:1-46

[74] Coomans A. Systematisch-ecologischonderzoek van de vrijlevendebodemnematoden in Belgie. De vrijlevendenematoden-fauna van weideland, I. Natuurwetenschap-pelijkTijdschrift. 1962;**43**:87-132

[75] Coomans A, Raski DJ. Aphanonchusintermediusn. g., n. sp. (Nemata: Araeolaimida). Nematologica. 1991;**37**:8-19

[76] Inglis WG. An outline classification of the phylum Nematoda. Australian Journal of Zoology. 1983;**31**:243-255

[77] Siddiqi MR. Tylenchida: parasites of plants and insects. CABI Publishing, Egham, UK. 2000. pp. 848

[78] Jairajpuri MS, Ahmad W. Dorylaimida - Free-living, predaceous and plant-parasitic nematodes. Delhi, India: Oxford and IBH Publishing Co; 1992. pp. 458

[79] Pushpalatha R. Entomopathogenic nematodes, farmers best friend! International Journal of Development Research. 2014;**4**(5):1088-1091

[80] Platt HM. Foreword. In The Phylogenetic Systematics of Free-living Nematodes. Lorenzen S, editor. pp. i–ii, The *Ray Society*, The Natural History Museum, Cromwell Road, *London*; 1994. pp. 383

[81] Örley L. Azanguillulidá kmagànrajza. (Monographie der Anguilluliden). Terméstzetrajz iFüzetek(Budapest). 1880;**4**:16-150

[82] Bongers T, Ferris H. Nematode community structureas a bioindicator inenvironmental monitoring. Trends Ecology. 1999;**14**(6):224

[83] Grewal PS, De Nardoe AB, Aguillera MM. Entomopathogenic Nematodes: Potential For Exploration and Use in South America. Neotropical Entomology. 2001;**30**(2):191-205

[84] Cobb NA. Antarctic marine free-living nematodes of the Shakelton expedition. Contributions to a Science of Nematology. 1914;3-33

[85] Caveness FE. A Glossary of Nematological Terms. Moor Plantation Press, Ibadan, Nigeria. 1964. pp. 68

Chapter 2

Methods and Tools Currently Used for the Identification of Plant Parasitic Nematodes

Regina Maria Dechechi Gomes Carneiro,
Fábia Silva de Oliveira Lima and
Valdir Ribeiro Correia

Additional information is available at the end of the chapter

http://dx.doi.org/10.5772/intechopen.69403

Abstract

Plant parasitic nematodes are one of the limiting factors for production of major crops worldwide. Overall, they cause an estimated annual crop loss of $78 billion worldwide and an average 10–15% crop yield losses. This imposes a challenge to sustainable production of food worldwide. Unsustainable cropping production with monocultures, intensive planting, and expansion of crops to newly opened areas has increased problems associated with nematodes. Thus, finding sustainable methods to control these pathogens is in current need. The correct diagnosis of nematode species is essential for choosing proper control methods and meaningful research. Morphology-based nematode taxonomy has been challenging due to intraspecific variation in characters. Alternatively, tools and methods based on biochemical and molecular markers have allowed successful diagnosis for a wide number of nematode species. Although these new methods have been useful due to their practical, fast, accuracy, and cost effective, the use of integrative diagnose, combining morphology, biochemical and molecular data is more appropriate when necessary to strength diagnose, define species boundaries, and to have a more suitable molecular database for nematode species. Here, we report a review on current methods and tools used to identify plant parasitic nematodes.

Keywords: diagnosis, isozyme, integrative, molecular, PCR, plant parasitic nematodes, root-knot nematodes

1. Introduction

Nematodes are diverse, microscopic multicellular animals comprising free living to plant parasitic species. They parasitize a wide range of plant species, including monocots and dicots and are one of the most limiting factors for major crops, causing an estimated annual crop loss of $78 billion worldwide and an average crop yield loss of 10–15% [1–3].

Reliable, fast, and proper nematode diagnosis and specimen identification are mandatory for choosing adequate management control strategies and for avoiding spreading of exotic nematodes in quarantine materials [4–7]. Nonetheless, nematodes are one of the most difficult organisms to be identified, either due to their small, microscopic sizes or due to the difficulties in observing key diagnostic characters/features under conventional light microscope [5, 7–10]. In addition, the differences of some of these morphological and morphometric characters are subtle, subjective, and have overlapping characters or show intraspecific variation which compromise proper identification or may lead to erroneous identity of the species [5, 10, 11]. Furthermore, nematode identification using classical morphology requires well trained and experienced nematode taxonomists which are in decline these days due to lack of interest of young scientists in classical taxonomy [10].

Currently, new methods and tools using biochemical and molecular approaches have been successfully used as diagnostic for plant parasitic nematodes [4, 6, 7, 10, 12–16]. Despite the feasibility and accuracy in using biochemical and molecular-based detection tools and methods these days, diagnoses based on morphology are still sufficient or are required in some specific cases. Thus, when possible, the use of integrative diagnostic/taxonomical approaches using morphological, biochemical, and molecular data may be more time consuming but overall may lead to a more accurate diagnosis of nematode species, especially for those cryptic or newly described species.

Diagnostic laboratory that provides testing for plant parasitic nematodes has been increasing in recent years due to increased occurrence, damage, and dissemination of plant parasitic nematodes, lack of proper control management strategies, and high population density of key nematode pests in agricultural systems [17]. The current withdrawal of most chemical nematicides from the market is direct consequence of their toxicity and side effects to environment and human health. Alternative means in controlling plant parasitic nematodes for a sustainable cropping system include the use of resistant cultivars, the use of non and poor hosts, crop rotation, crop succession, and biological control [5]. However, accurate and fast identification of nematodes to species and subspecies levels is mandatory not only to be successful in choosing a proper management strategy but also for studying their genetic and biological variability or to avoid global spread of exotic and quarantine pathogens [4, 6, 7, 18, 19].

The goal of this chapter is to report a literature review of methods and tools to identify the most common genera of plant parasitic nematodes and its use to other nematode species as well.

2. Morphology-based diagnosis of nematodes

Nematode diagnosis and taxonomy have traditionally relied on morphological and anatomical characters using light microscopy. Lately, despite the increased interest in molecular diagnosis, due to its feasibility which allow quick and easy identification of specimens and allow researchers and extensions folks to use these techniques for routine use [10], classical taxonomy using reliable and nonoverlapping morphological characters is still an important tool for the identification of nematodes mainly for the following reasons: (i) it allows a clear link between function and morphological aspects of the specimen analyzed; (ii) it is still a method that provides fast results; (iii) it is suitable for quantitative evaluations; (iv) it is cheaper; and (v) it is used for population surveys of plant parasitic nematodes with the objective to recommend management control strategies [10].

Other disadvantage in using classical taxonomy, besides the drawback of obscure morphological characters afore mentioned, the preparation of nematode specimens for classical identification, may result in modifications of the nematode, which may be difficult in its proper identification. For instance, much of the nematode body composition is proteins and fats, which undergo immediate coagulation or other alteration during the processing of the specimens, due to the use of substances such as sucrose, formaldehyde, glycerin, and the heating to which they are normally subjected during fixation [20]. In this way, specimens after being extracted, killed, fixed, and mounted on microscopic preparations, frequently present artifacts that make it difficult to locate external or internal structures of diagnostic value, or even produce characteristics that are not natural [20].

According to Inserra et al. [20], other disadvantages of light microscopy, in relation to other methods (electron microscopy, isozyme electrophoresis, and molecular methods), are as follows: the need for specimens in excellent preservation conditions; some characteristics of diagnostic value show high intraspecific variation, reason for the need for more than safe examination, need for abundant and updated scientific literature, the need for a taxonomist to be deepened in taxonomical studies, who probably would be a specialist in only a few groups of nematodes; several morphological and morphometric characteristics of diagnostic value are modified by environmental factors, such as geographic location, host plant species, host plant mineral nutrition, and light. However, the main disadvantage is that microscopic examination is not sufficient for identifying morphological characters that are extremely difficult to observe [20]. Thus, using integrative diagnostic approaches with more than one diagnostic method is less prone to errors.

3. Morphological and biochemical identification of *Meloidogyne* spp.

Root-knot nematodes (RKNs), *Meloidogyne* spp., are the most aggressive, damaging, and economically important group of plant parasitic nematodes infecting important crops worldwide. Currently, about 97 *Meloidogyne* spp. have been described [5], of which *M. arenaria, M. incognita, M. javanica*, and *M. hapla* represent up to 95% of RKN in cultivated soils.

This group of nematodes is highly diverse, showing a continuum of diversity in terms of cytogenetics (variable chromosomes numbers with aneuploidy and polyploidy states), mode of reproduction (ranging from amphimixis to obligatory-mitotic parthenogenesis), specialization in parasitism, species complexes, cryptic species, interspecific hybridization, and broad host ranges [4, 6, 7, 18, 21]. Overall, this high level of diversity contributes to an extremely complex relationship with their hosts that lead to highly successful parasitism. For example, the three major *Meloidogyne* spp. (i.e., *M. incognita, M. javanica*, and *M. arenaria*) are highly polyphagous, infecting more than 3000 plant species [5].

Diagnosis of *Meloidogyne* spp. has traditionally relied on the characterization of female perineal patterns and morphometrics. However, since these morphological characters overlap in some RKN species (e.g., in *M. paranaensis, M. konaensis*, and *M. enterolobii*), misidentification of species using morphology as the only criteria is often frequent [22, 23].

The morphology of female perineal patterns has been a character most frequently used in several laboratories for the identification of *Meloidogyne* species, a character located in the posterior body region of adult females. This area comprises the vulva-anus area (perineum), tail terminus, phasmids, lateral lines, and surrounding cuticular striae. Preparation of perineal patterns for the observation and identification of *Meloidogyne* spp. has been covered by different authors. A more detailed account on root-knot nematode perineal pattern development was given by Karssen [23]. **Figure 1** summarizes the perineal patterning for 12 major *Meloidogyne* species that are considered important to major crops [5].

For many years, the identification of *Meloidogyne* spp. has been relied upon the characterization of adult female perineal pattern and the use of several morphometric and morphological features of juveniles. To these characters were added features of male (although they are rarely seen), such as the form of the labial region, including annulation, and the form of stylet and basal knobs. However, with increasing numbers of described species, the value of many of these characters, themselves showing often large intraspecific variation, was eroded almost to the point where robust identification tended to involve a fair measure of serendipity. As an example, what may be termed the *incognita*-type of perineal pattern is now known to occur in a substantial number of species, some of which were commonly misidentified as *M. incognita*.

As an alternative to morphological identification of *Meloidogyne* spp., esterase patterning has been used for diagnosing *Meloidogyne* spp. from a wide range of samples and has been proved to be species-specific for a number of species [13, 24, 25]. *Meloidogyne* spp., isozyme electrophoresis patterning has discriminated all of these otherwise cryptic species, however, this technique is restricted to females [24]. Examples of esterase patterning for major *Meloidogyne* spp. are shown in **Figure 2**.

One of the earliest examples of the use of isozyme phenotypes to distinguish *Meloidogyne* spp. was given by Esbenshade and Triantaphyllou [25], who reported esterase patterns for 16 *Meloidogyne* species, with the most common phenotypes being A2 and A3 (*M. arenaria*), H1 (*M. hapla*), I1 (*M. incognita*), and J3 (*M. javanica*). In landmark surveys for *Meloidogyne* spp. using isozyme [12, 25] study, approximately 300 populations originate from 65 countries and several continents. In later surveys, Carneiro et al. [22] found 18 esterase phenotypes among 111 populations of *Meloidogyne* spp. from Brazil and other South American countries. Isozymes continue to be widely used for diagnosis of *Meloidogyne* spp. despite some limitations. Nonetheless, isozyme phenotyping has been used for a large number of species [6]. Schematic diagrams of isozyme patterns based on surveys, including those conducted in the international *Meloidogyne* project have been published [8, 12, 22, 25] and provide important references.

Several isozyme systems have been used, nonetheless, carboxylesterase/esterase EST proved to be the most useful in discriminating *Meloidogyne* species. Others, such as malate dehydrogenase (MDH), are also often included to confirm species identification [25]. Enzyme phenotypes

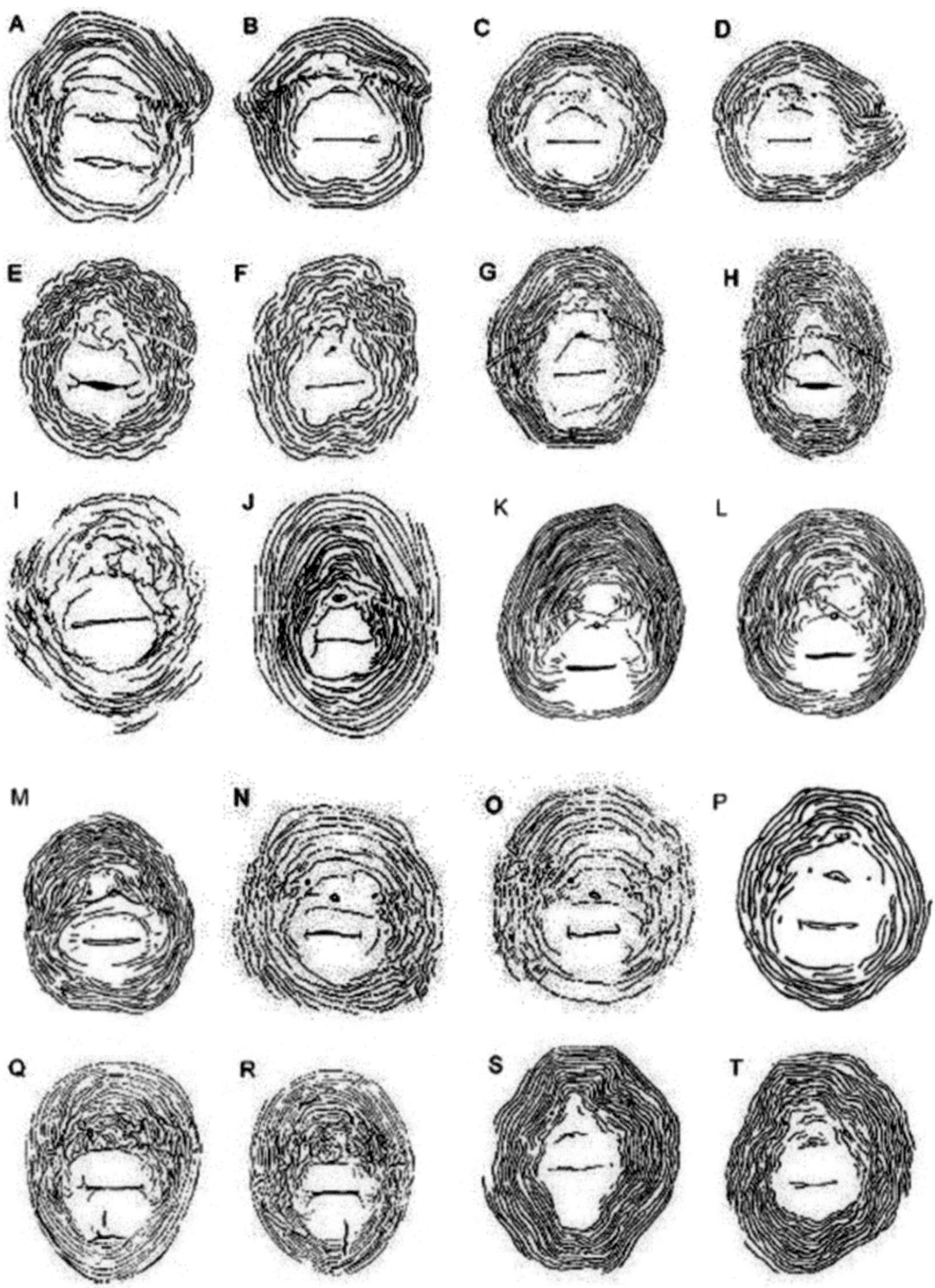

Figure 1. Comparison of perineal patterns for 12 major *Meloidogyne* spp. A, B: *M. arenaria*; C, D: *M. hapla*; E, F: *M. incognita*; G, H: *M. javanica*; I: *M. acronea*; J: *M. chitwoodi*; K, L: *M. enterolobii*; M: *M. ethiopica*; N, O: *M. exigua*; P: *M. fallax*; Q, R: *M. graminicola*; S, T: *M. paranaensis*. Drawings not to scale [5].

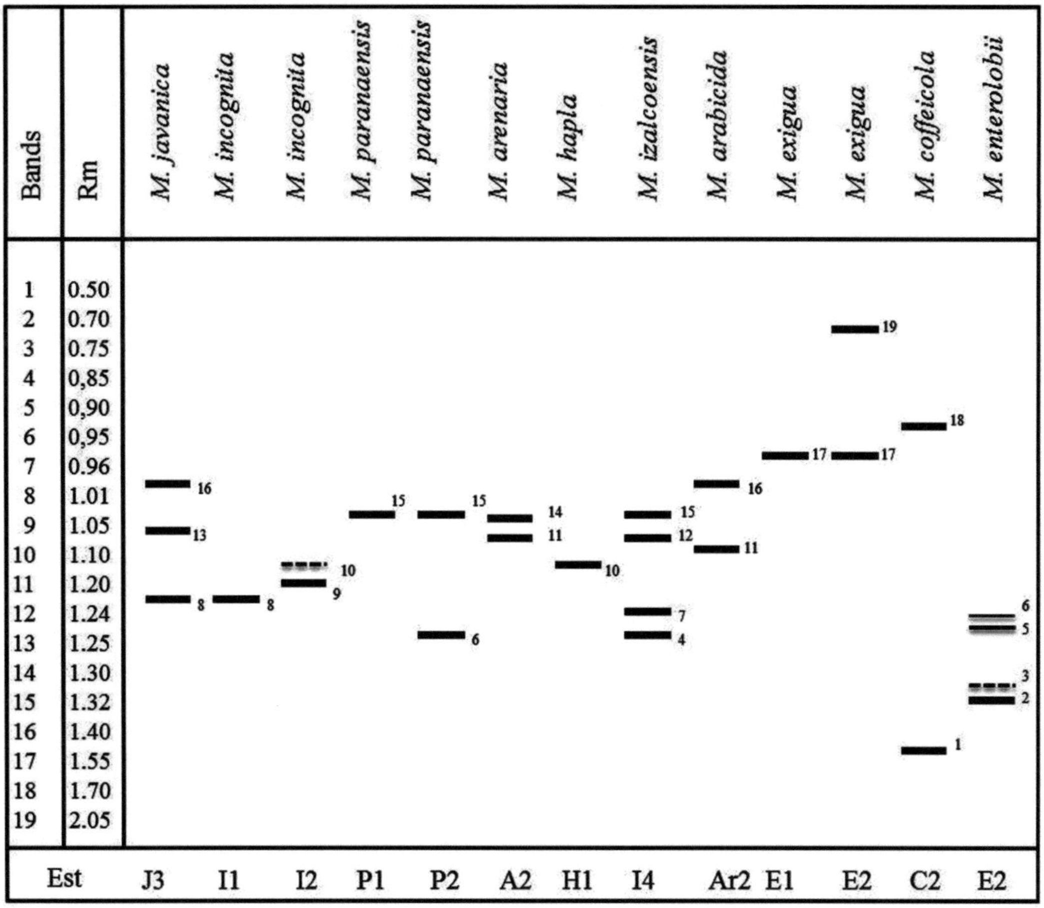

Figure 2. Esterase phenotypes (Est) of major *Meloidogyne* spp. associated with coffee. Rm = ratio of migration in relation to the fast band of *M. javanica*. Dotted lines indicate weak bands [24].

patterning are designated, indicating the *Meloidogyne* species that each specifies and the number of bands detected. Phenotypes with the same number of bands are differentiated by small letters [12, 25]. Enzyme patterns are usually compared with a known standard, with *M. javanica* being frequently used to determine migration distances among bands. Isozymes are used primarily with female egg-laying stage, using single individuals. Miniaturization and automation of the electrophoresis systems and the use of precast polyacrylamide gels (i.e., PhastSytem, Pharmacia Ltd, Uppsala, Sweden) have made isozyme phenotyping a widely used technique in most labs [22, 23, 25]. Classical electrophoresis methods using vertical and horizontal systems were also described in details in Refs. [13, 25], respectively.

Aside from the initial equipment cost, the consumables required are relatively inexpensive and isozymes have been often used for field surveys, diagnosis, as well as with routine screening of glasshouse cultures to assure species stability and pure cultures. The relative stability of isozyme phenotypes within *Meloidogyne* species makes them an attractive system, although there are some drawbacks. For instance, the occurrence of intraspecific variants and the difficulty in resolving the same esterase phenotype between species (e.g., *M. exigua* vs. *M. naasi*) have required the use of an additional enzyme system (e.g., MDH) to confirm species identity. In addition, weak bands on the polyacrylamide gel may need to use a larger number of females per well (e.g., *M. exigua*) [22]. For some species, there are more than one esterase phenotype for a same species—e.g., *M. javanica* (J3, J2, and J2a), *M. incognita* (I1, I2, and S2), *M. arenaria* (A2 and A1), *M. exigua* (E1, E2, and E3), and *M. paranaensis* (P1 and P2) [8, 9, 26].

In surveys with the objective to study *Meloidogyne* biodiversity and nature conservancy, isozymes are a convenient first stage in species identification and have enabled the study of species diversity and frequency of a particular species, as well as their abundance. Females recovered after allowing multiplication of field samples on a generally susceptible host such as tomato (*Solanum lycopersicum*) can be tested for their isozyme phenotypes and the associated egg mass reserved for further characterization, if necessary [22]. Thus, novel isozyme phenotypes have been frequently found in these surveys in conserved areas, overall adding to the understanding of species ecology and biogeography of *Meloidogyne* spp. The Esbenshade and Triantaphyllou [25] listed Est F1 as an undescribed phenotype from Brazil; Later, *M. paranaensis* was described showing this phenotype [27]. In addition, Carneiro et al. [22] listed the patterns Est K3, Est Y3, and Est L3 as atypical esterase phenotypes; later, *M. ethiopica* and *M. inornata* were identified showing these new esterase patterns [8–9]. Recently, *M. luci* (Est L3) was described as a new species [28]. The phenotype Est Sa4 (Rm 73.5, 78.0, 53.0, 59.0), a new esterase phenotype from coffee in Central America, was later described as *M. izalcoensis* [29].

Isozyme electrophoretic profiles, often using esterase (EST) and malate dehydrogenase (MDH), have been established for a number of species [6] and can provide a useful routine diagnostic test particularly for morphologically variable species, such as *M. arenaria.* This species showed different profiles and high intraspecific variability, it may be an indication of the existence of species swam. Recently, the Est phenotype A3 of *M. arenaria* was identified as *M. morocciensis* [9].

Although isozyme electrophoresis is currently one of the best methods for *Meloidogyne* spp. diagnosis, it seems likely that DNA-based methods and tools will soon usurp this method for many applications where finer resolution, particularly of intraspecific variation, is paramount [6]. Nonetheless, the use of an integrative diagnosis, combining more than one approach, such as morphology, morphometrics, biochemical, and molecular data is less prone to error and could be used when possible.

4. Molecular diagnosis of plant parasitic nematodes

Since the development of polymerase chain reaction (PCR) and the vast amount of genetic data generated with DNA sequencing, molecular-based detection tools have been widely developed and successfully used for the diagnosis of plant parasitic nematodes. Molecular-based detection tools have the following advantages as compared with other methods, (i) can be used in a high throughput manner, (ii) DNA information can be acquired easily with the vast amount of databases and sequencing information, (iii) are cheap, fast, and accurate, (iv) DNA markers are independent of phenotypic variation and developmental stage of the nematode [14].

DNA-based markers have been proved reliable and have allowed diagnosis and description of new species for several groups of nematodes, including key genera such as *Meloidogyne, Pratylenchus, Globodera,* and *Heterodera* [4, 6, 7, 10, 18, 30–32]. DNA-based detection tools make excellent methods of nematode diagnosis since they are simple, accurate, and fast [6, 7] and can be used with a wide range of sample types, including host tissue, eggs, egg masses, soil extracts, and fixed samples [16].

Nowadays, most labs worldwide are commonly using molecular methods to diagnose nematodes since cost associated with reagents and equipment are affordable and there has been a crescent interest in molecular taxonomy by young scientists [10, 16]. These methods have been used ordinary and are sensitive enough to detect individual nematodes from complex types of samples, including soil samples and species mixtures in the field [21, 33–35]. Some limitations of molecular-based detection tools include problems associated with optimization and validation of tools and methods, DNA extraction protocols, conditions of samples (i.e., quarantine specimens), amount of target DNA in a sample, cross contamination, false positive and negative results, which overall should be used carefully as to not compromise the ultimate result of diagnosis [16].

4.1. Ribosomal DNA

A vast amount of examples of nematode diagnosis has mostly been based on amplification of target DNA by PCR using species-specific primers. PCR-based detection methods have revolutionized the area of diagnostics of nematodes and have been used due to improved sensitivity, specificity, speed, relatively ease to perform, and cost effectiveness compared with other diagnostic procedures [4, 6, 7, 10, 18]. One of the approaches to design DNA-based markers that can aided diagnosis of nematodes has been based usually on conserved regions in the ribosomal DNA (rDNA) cistron, i.e., the external transcribed spacer (ETS), internal transcribed spacers 1 and 2 (ITS1 and ITS2), and the intergenic spacer regions 1 and 2 (IGS1 and IGS2) [7]. Schematic representation of these genetic regions is shown in **Figure 3**.

In this way, sequences that are divergent among nematode species and conserved within several isolates of a same species make ideal target for designing species-specific primers [7]. Ribosomal DNA regions have been very suitable for choosing a target marker since they are

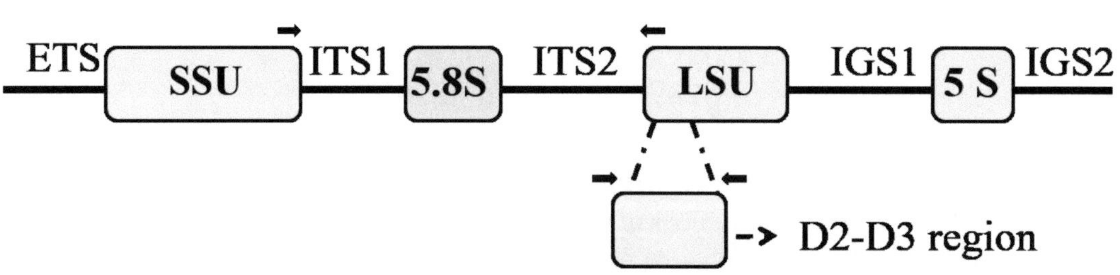

Figure 3. Schematic representation of nuclear rRNA genes in eukaryotic cells. SSU = 18S—small subunit; LSU = 28S—large subunit; ETS—external transcribed spacer region; ITS1 and ITS2—internal transcribed spacers; IGS1 and IGS2—intergenic spacer regions; arrows indicate possible starting point for primer amplification. Open box indicates the D2-D3 expansion segments for the 28S rRNA.

multicopy genes and provide sequences with enough variation that can be used for diagnosis and phylogenetic relationships among species [7].

4.2. Mitochondrial and satellite DNA

Diagnostics of nematodes have also been based on other genomic target regions such as mitochondrial DNA (mtDNA). Mitochondrial DNA genomes are relatively small circular molecules ranging from 12 to 20 kilobases [7, 36]. Divergences in mtDNA sequences due to insertions, deletions, and accelerated ratio of mutations compared with nuclear DNA [7] have provided target markers suitable for discriminating nematode species [37–39].

Satellite DNAs (satDNAs) are highly repeated tandem arrays of short sequences ranging from 70 to 2000 bp. It has different signature sequences, copy numbers, length, and polymorphic regions that can be explored to find species-specific markers [6, 7]. Such PCR-based detection using satDNA markers in nematode diagnosis has been reported by several labs [7, 40, 41] and represents a target option for designing diagnostic primers.

4.3. RFLP, AFLP, RAPD, SCAR

One of the first methods used to differentiate nematode species was restriction fragment length polymorphism (RFLP), a method that uses restriction enzymes to digest whole genomic DNA or an amplified segment of it to generate DNA banding patterns according to divergences in sequences among isolates [7, 42]. This technique can also be coupled with DNA hybridization with radioactive or nonradioactive labeled probes [7]. Although being effective in differentiating nematode isolates, this method is less used nowadays due to technical complexity and the need for a large amount of target DNA, which usually requires preculturing of nematode populations [6, 7].

Alternatively, species-specific primers have been designed from sequences randomly scattered throughout nematode genomes, e.g., DNA band obtained from random amplified polymorphic DNA (RAPD) or amplified fragment length polymorphism (AFLP) gels, with posterior cloning and sequencing of bands differential across related species and their conversion into species-specific sequence characterized amplified region (SCAR) markers [21, 43–46]. SCAR-based markers and rDNA-based specific primers have been used to diagnose nematodes with either conventional or real-time PCR (q-PCR) [6, 7, 10].

Numerous primers and approaches used for diagnosis of nematodes using conventional and quantitative PCR were designed based on several target regions in the nematode genome (e.g., SCAR, rDNA, ITS, D2-D3 segment, IGS, among others). **Table 1** summarizes some of these strategies used in some main studies.

In particular, successful SCAR markers have been developed for diagnosing some of the major tropical *Meloidogyne* spp. associated with important crops such as coffee, guava, and grapevine, including *M. arenaria* [43], *M. incognita* [21], *M. paranaensis, M. exigua* [21], *M. enterolobii* [44], *M. arabicida, M. izalcoensis* [45], and *M. ethiopica* [46] (see a complete list of references for species-specific primers in **Table 1**). These primers were validated in several population studies,

Nematode species	Target region	Method	References
***Meloidogyne* spp.**			
M. arabicida and *M. izalcoensis*	SCAR*	PCR	[45]
M. arenaria	SCAR	PCR	[43]
M. chitwoodi	IGS	PCR	[47]
	SCAR	PCR	[48]
M. exigua	SCAR	PCR	[21]
M. enterolobii	mtDNA	PCR	[49]
	SCAR	PCR	[44]
M. ethiopica	SCAR	PCR	[46]
M. fallax	IGS	PCR	[47]
	SCAR	PCR	[48]
M. graminis	ITS	PCR	[11]
M. hapla	satDNA	PCR	[50]
M. hapla	SCAR	PCR	[48]
	IGS	PCR	[51]
M. incognita	SCAR	PCR	[43]
	SCAR	PCR	[21]
M. javanica	SCAR	PCR	[43]
	SCAR	PCR	[52]
M. marylandi	28S D2-D3	PCR	[11]
M. naasi	ITS	PCR	[52]
M. naasi	28S D2-D3	PCR	[11]
M. paranaensis	SCAR	PCR	[21]
Other parasitic nematodes			
Bursaphelencus xylophilus	satDNA	PCR	[53]
B. xylophilus	satDNA	qPCR	[54]
B. xylophilus	heat shock protein	qPCR	[55]
Ditylenchus destructor D. dipsaci	rDNA	PCR/qPCR	[56]
H. glycines	rDNA	qPCR	[57]
H. schachtii	ITS	PCR	[58]
H. glycines	SCAR	qPCR	[59]
Pratylenchus penetrans	rDNA	qPCR	[60]

*SCAR—sequence characterized amplified region; IGS—intergenic spacer region; ITS—internal transcribed spacer; mtDNA—mitochondrial DNA; satDNA—satellite DNA; PCR—polymerase chain reaction; qPCR—quantitative real-time PCR.

Table 1. Species-specific primers for diagnosis of selected plant parasitic nematodes.

using DNA from a single juvenile (J2), or in multiplex PCR reactions containing mixtures of species, and have become an excellent practical diagnostic kit for certain crops-associated *Meloidogyne* spp. [8, 21, 45, 46]. Interestingly, [61] established a diagnostic key for the identification of seven RKN species, i.e., *M. incognita, M. javanica, M. arenaria, M. enterolobii, M. hapla, M. chitwoodi,* and *M. fallax* using a combination of IGS PCR, SCAR markers, and RAPD profiling.

4.4. qPCR and barcoding

Quantitative PCR (q-PCR) is a technique that amplifies and quantifies nucleic acids simultaneously. Its advantage over conventional PCR is that it is fast, sensitive and does not need post-amplification processing of samples normally seen in conventional PCR, which can lead to false results in some cases, reviewed in Refs. [7, 10]. As new genomic sequences become available for plant parasitic nematodes, there have been a vast number of examples of this approach to detect and quantify nematodes from a wide range of samples, including greenhouse, field experiments, ecological studies, experiments with plant-nematode interactions, and virus load in nematode vector and are being used as the advantage to be fast, accurate and to be applicable in high throughput processing systems of large number of samples, reviewed in Ref. [10]. Application of q-PCR in nematode diagnosis using rDNA target or other marker has been showed for major nematode species, including *M. incognita, M. chitwoodi, M. fallax, M. javanica, Bursaphelenchus xylophilus, Globodera rostochiensis,* and *G. pallida*. For a complete list of nematodes, see Ref. [10].

The concept of DNA barcode for nematode taxonomy has been employed in Ref. [62] and is related to a DNA sequence of a particular region in the genome as a mean to give unique signature (barcode) for the identification of nematode species [7]. Although theoretically sounds, this approach has not been widely accepted since there has not been an unique DNA locus that can define the limits of species boundary and be used as universal identification of nematodes, besides the missing link of DNA barcode approach with classical taxonomy which has shown clear methods for species-level resolution [7, 14].

4.5. Soil PCR

Lately, there has been increased interest of labs to perform molecular diagnosis of nematodes directly from soil samples without the need to extract the target nematode species, a strategy commonly used for communities of bacteria and fungi [7]. There are available commercial kits for the direct extraction of nematode DNA from soil extracts and has been successfully employed in some labs. Alternatively, nematodes can be extracted from soil samples using conventional methods such as Baerman funnel, Whitehead tray or other method can be pooled for DNA extraction using commercial kits or other ordinary DNA extraction method. This strategy has been used by several authors and has been proved reliable and time saving [33, 34]. Nonetheless, there are drawbacks associated with this strategy, including underestimation of nematodes due to their uneven distribution in the soil, the limited amount of soil sample used for DNA extraction in commercial kits and the cost associated with sample processing [7].

Alternatively, a method to enrich nematode from soil extract using antibody-based capture was proposed by Chen et al. [63]; however, its use as routine diagnosis in labs needs to be analyzed.

5. Concluding remarks

The accurate identification of nematodes to species and subspecies levels is essential for their control and is a prerequisite to meaningful research. Many nematode species are easily identified based on distinct morphological characters and restricted host ranges. Several species are difficult to identify due to their similarity to other species or poor taxonomic descriptions. The difficulty in identifying nematodes species may result from morphological variations within and between populations from a same species.

Problems in the morphological identification of nematodes species, such as large number of described species within a specific group, e.g., as to compare several observed characters seen by light or scanning microscopy, and lack of apparent differences in a certain feature between species, e.g., perineal patterns, have encouraged much interest in the use of biochemical and molecular techniques as routine methods for the identification of nematodes. Biochemical and molecular methods used for the identification of nematodes are now widely used and are essential for diagnosis of a wide range of plant parasitic nematodes.

A clear understanding of species boundaries and adequate sampling of known species across their geographic areas are lacking in several regions and important crops. The future prospects in nematode taxonomy and diagnostics are dependent on molecular-based methods and tools that will discriminate not only at the species level but also at the level of host races, thereby opening up opportunities for more focused management strategies. Such techniques offer the possibility of rapid, unequivocal diagnostics and should help resolve the present problems associated with relatively morphologically conserved organisms that reproduce, for the most part, parthenogenetically, as is the case of *Meloidogyne* spp.

As for the case of taxonomy for *Meloidogyne* spp., once such molecular techniques are widely employed, no doubt the number of current nominal species will be shown to be junior synonyms, while others, conversely, will be shown to be species complexes, possibly of sibling species. It seems likely that molecular methods will replace isozymes as the preferred diagnostic tool for *Meloidogyne* spp. because of their inherently higher resolution and the opportunity to develop DNA chips for rapid and reliable field identification.

Molecular tools will also enhance our understanding of phylogenetic relatedness of nematodes and its relationship with other plant parasitic nematodes. Although nucleic acids-based detection techniques have been useful in diagnosing nematode species due to their high throughput characteristics, fast, sensitivity and cost effectiveness, the use of integrative diagnose approaches for nematode identification, combining morphology, biochemical and molecular data are more appropriate when necessary to strength nematode identification, define species boundaries, and to have a more suitable molecular database for nematode species.

A vast amount of genetic data are becoming available with nematode genome sequencing, which provides tools to perform comparative genomes and finds target DNA regions that can be used as diagnostic marker.

Molecular-based detection tools and methods are aimed to aid nematode taxonomy and should not totally exclude classical taxonomy approaches since in some cases, they must be complementary for accurate diagnosis.

Author details

Regina Maria Dechechi Gomes Carneiro[1], Fábia Silva de Oliveira Lima[2] and Valdir Ribeiro Correia[2]*

*Address all correspondence to: valdir.correia@ifto.edu.br

1 Embrapa Recursos Genéticos e Biotecnologia, Brasília, DF, Brazil

2 Instituto Federal de Educação, Ciência e Tecnologia do Tocantins, Dianópolis, TO, Brazil

References

[1] Maggenti, A. General Nematology. 1st ed. New York: Springer-Verlag; 1981. p. 372. DOI: 10.1007/978-1-4612-5938-1

[2] Barker K. Introduction and synopsis of advancement in nematodes. In: Barker KR, Pederson GA, Windham GL, editors. Plant Nematode Interactions. 1st ed. Madison, WI: ASA, CSSA, SSSA; 1998. pp. 1-20

[3] Hugot JP, Baujard P, Morand S. Biodiversity in helminthes and nematodes as a field of study. Nematology. 2001;**3**:199-208

[4] Blok VC. Achievements in and future prospects for molecular diagnosis of plant parasitic nematodes. Canadian Journal of Plant Pathology. 2005;**27**:176-185

[5] Hunt D, Handoo Z. Taxonomy, identification and principal species. In: Perry RN, Moens M, Star JL, editors. Root Knot Nematodes. 1st ed. London: CABI International; 2009. pp. 55-88

[6] Blok VC, Powers TO. Biochemical and molecular identification. In: Perry RN, Moens M, Star J, editors. Root Knot Nematodes. 1st ed. London: CABI International; 2009. pp. 98-112

[7] Castagnone-Sereno P. Molecular tools for diagnosis. In: Jones J, Gheisen G, Fenoll C, editors. Genomics and Molecular Genetics of Plant Nematode Interactions. 1st ed. New York: Springer; 2011. pp. 443-464

[8] Carneiro RMDG, Tigano MS, Randig O, Almeida MRA, Sarah JL. Identification and genetic diversity of *Meloidogyne* spp. (Tylenchida: Meloidogynidae) on coffee from Brazil, Central America and Hawaii. Nematology. 2004;**6**:287-298

[9] Carneiro RMDG, Dos Santos MFA, Almeida MRA, Mota FC, Gomes ACMM, Tigano MS. Diversity of *Meloidogyne arenaria* using morphological, cytological and molecular approaches. Nematology. 2008;**10**:819-834

[10] Oliveira CMG, Monteiro AR, Blok VC. Morphological and molecular diagnostics for plant parasitic nematodes: Working together to get the identification done. Tropical Plant Pathology. 2011;**36**(2):065-073

[11] Ye W, Zeng Y, Kerns J. Molecular characterisation and diagnosis of root-knot nematodes (*Meloidogyne* spp.) from Turfgrasses in North Carolina, USA. PLoS One. 2015; **10**(11):e0143556. DOI: 10.1371/journal.pone.0143556

[12] Esbenshade PR, Triantaphyllou AC. Isozyme phenotypes for identification of *Meloidogyne* species. Journal of Nematology. 1990;**22**:10-15

[13] Carneiro RMDG, Almeida MRA. Técnica de eletroforese usada no estudo de enzimas dos nematoides das galhas para identificação de espécies. Nematologia Brasileira. 2001;**25**:35-44

[14] Abebe E, Mekete T, Thomas WK. A critique of current methods in nematode taxonomy. African Journal of Biotechnology. 2011;**10**(3):312-323. DOI: 105899/AJB10.1473

[15] Holterman MM, Oggenfuss M, Frey JE, Kiewnik S. Evaluation of high-resolution melting curve analysis as a new tool for root knot nematode diagnostics. Phytopathology. 2012;**160**:59-66

[16] Nega A. Review on nematode molecular diagnostics: From bands to barcode. Journal of Biology, Agriculture and Healthcare. 2014;**4**(27):1-26

[17] Lima FSO, Santos GR, Nogueira SR, Santos PRR, Correa VR. Population dynamics of the root lesion nematode *Pratylenchus brachyurus* in soybean fields in Tocantins state and its effect to soybean yield. Nematropica. 2015;**45**(2):170-177

[18] Powers TO. Nematode molecular diagnostics. Annual Review of Phytopathology. 2004; **42**:367-383

[19] Skantar AM, Carta LK. Amplification of Hsp90 homologs from plant parasitic nematodes using degenerate primers and ramped annealing PCR. Journal of Nematology. 2000;**29**:1182-1186

[20] Inserra R, Duncan LW, Troccoli A, Santos J, Kaplan D, Volvas N. *Pratylenchus Jaehni* n. sp. from citrus in Brazil and its relationship with *P. coffeae* and *P. loosi*. Nematology. 2001;**3**:653-665

[21] Randig O, Bongiovanni M, Carneiro RMDG, Castagnone-Sereno P. Genetic diversity of root knot nematodes from Brazil and development of SCAR markers specific for the coffee-damaging species. Genome. 2002;**45**:862-870

[22] Carneiro RMDG, Almeida MRA, Queneherve P. Enzyme phenotypes of *Meloidogyne* spp populations. Nematology. 2000;**2**:645-654

[23] Karssen G. The Plant Parasitic Nematode Genus *Meloidogyne* Goeldi 1892 (Tylenchida) in Europe. 1st ed. Leiden: Brill; 2002. p. 157

[24] Carneiro RMDG, Cofcewics ET. Taxonomy of coffee parasitic root knot nematodes, *Meloidogyne* spp. In: Souza RM, editor. Plant Parasitic Nematodes of Coffee. 1st ed. Netherland: Springer Netherlands; 2008. pp. 87-122. DOI: 10.1007/978-1-4020-8720-2_6

[25] Esbenshade PR, Triantaphyllou AC. Use of enzyme phenotypes for identification of *Meloidogyne* species. Journal of Nematology. 1985;**17**(1):6-20

[26] Muniz MFS, Campos VP, Castagnone-Sereno P, Castro JMC, Almeida MRA, Carneiro RMDG. Diversity of *Meloidogyne exigua* (Tylenchida: Meloidogynidae) populations from coffee and rubber tree. Nematology. 2008;**10**:897-910

[27] Carneiro RMDG, Carneiro RG, Abrantes IMO, Santos MFA, Almeida MRA. *Meloidogyne paranaensis* n. sp (Nemata: Meloidogynidae), a root knot nematode parasitising coffee in Brazil. Journal of Nematology. 1996;**28**(2):177-189

[28] Carneiro RMDG, Correa VR, Almeida RMA, Gomes ACMM, Deimi AM, Castagnone-Sereno P, Karssen G. *Meloidogyne luci* n. sp. a root knot nematode parasitising different crops in Brazil, Chile and Iran. Nematology. 2014;**16**(3):1-13

[29] Carneiro RMDG, Almeida MRA, Gomes ACMM, Hernandez A. *Meloidogyne izalcoensis* n. sp. (Nematode: Meloidogynidae), a root knot nematode parasitizing coffee in El Salvador. Nematology. 2005;**76**(6):819-832

[30] Shields R, Fleming CC, Stratford R. Identification of potato cyst nematodes using the Polymerase Chain Reaction. Fundamental and Applied Nematology. 1996;**19**:167-173

[31] Powers TO, Todd TC, Burnell AM, Murray PCB, Fleming CC, Szalanski AL, Adams BA, Harris TS. The rDNA internal transcribed spacer region as a taxonomic marker for nematodes. Journal of Nematology. 1997;**29**:441-450

[32] Subbotin SA, Halford PD, Warry A, Perry RN. Variations in ribosomal DNA sequences and phylogeny of *Globodera* parasitizing solanaceous plantas. Nematology. 2000;**2**:591-604

[33] Holeva R. Molecular differentiation of Trichodorid nematodes and functional studies of the transmission [thesis]. Dundee: University of Dundee; 2004

[34] Machado ACZ, Ferraz LCCB, Oliveira CMG. Development of species-specific reverse primer for the molecular diagnostic of *Pratylenchus brachyurus*. Nematropica. 1997;**37**:249-257

[35] Yan GP, Smiley RW, Okubara PA, Skantar A, Easley SA, Sheedy JG, Thompson AL. Detection and discrimination of *Pratylenchus neglectus* and *P. thornei* in DNA extracts from soil. Plant Disease. 2008;**92**:1480-1487

[36] Brown WM. The mitochondrial genome of animals. In: Macintyre RJ, editors. Molecular Evolutionary Genetics. 1st ed. New York: Plenum; 1985. pp. 95-130

[37] Powers TO, Harris TS. A polymerase chain reaction method for the detection of five major *Meloidogyne* species. Journal of Nematology. 1993;**23**:1-6

[38] Stanton J, Hugall A, Moritz C. Nucleotide polymorphisms and an improved PCR-based mtDNA diagnostic for parthenogenetic root-knot nematodes (*Meloidogyne* spp). Fundamental and Applied Nematology. 1997;**20**:261-268

[39] Jeyaprakash A, Tigano MS, Brito J, Carneiro RMDG, Dickson DW. Differentiation of *Meloidogyne floridensis* from *M. arenaria* using high-fidelity PCR amplified mitochondrial AT- rich sequences. Nematropica. 2006;**36**:1-12

[40] Castagnone-Sereno P, Esparrago G, Abad P, Leroy F, Bongiovanni M. Satellite DNA as a target for PCR-specific detection of the plant-parasitic nematode *Meloidogyne hapla*. Current Genetics. 1995;**28**:566-570

[41] Randig O, Deau F, dos Santos MFA, Tigano MS, Carneiro RMDG, Castagnone-Sereno P. A novel species-specific satellite DNA family in the invasive root-knot nematode *Meloidogyne mayaguensis* and its potential use for diagnostics. European Journal of Plant Pathology. 2009;**125**:485-495

[42] Curran J, Baillie DL, Webster JM. Use of genomic DNA restriction fragment length polymorphism to identify nematode species. Parasitology. 1985;**90**:137-144

[43] Zijlstra C, Donkers-Venne DTHM, Fargette M. Identification of *Meloidogyne incognita, M. javanica* and *M. arenaria* using sequence characterised amplified region (SCAR) based PCR assays. Nematology. 2000;**2**:847-883

[44] Tigano M, Siqueira K, Castagnone-Sereno P, Mulet K, Queiroz P, Santos M, Teixeira C, Almeida M, Silva J, Carneiro RMDG. Genetic diversity of the root-knot nematode *Meloidogyne enterolobii* and development of a SCAR marker for this guava-damaging species. Plant Pathology. 2010;**59**(6):1054-1061

[45] Correa VR, Santos MFA, Almeida MRA, Peixoto JR, Castagnone-Sereno P, Carneiro RMDG. Species-specific DNA markers for identification of two root-knot nematodes of coffee: *Meloidogyne arabicida* and *M. izalcoensis*. European Journal of Plant Pathology. 2013;**137**:305-313

[46] Correa VR, Mattos VS, Almeida MRA, Santos MFA, Tigano MS, Castagnone-Sereno P, Carneiro RMDG. Genetic diversity of the root-knot nematode *Meloidogyne ethiopica* and development of a species-specific SCAR marker for its diagnosis. Plant Pathology. 2014;**63**(2):476-483

[47] Petersen DJ, Zijlstra C, Wishart J, Blok V, Vrain TC. Specific probes efficiently distinguish root-knot nematode species using signature sequences in the ribosomal intergenic spacer. Fundamental and Applied Nematology. 1997;**20**:619-626

[48] Zijlstra C. Identification of *Meloidogyne chitwoodi, M. fallax* and *M. hapla* based on SCAR-PCR: A powerful way of enabling reliable identification of populations or individuals that share common traits. European Journal of Plant Pathology. 2000;**106**:283-290

[49] Blok VC, Wishart J, Fargette M, Berthier K, Phillips MS. Mitochondrial differences distinguishing *Meloidogyne mayaguensis* from the major species of tropical root-knot nematodes. Nematology. 2002;**4**:773-781

[50] Piotte C, Castagnone-Sereno P, Bongiovanni M, Dalmasso A, Abad P. Analysis of a satellite DNA from *Meloidogyne hapla* and its use as a diagnostic probe. Phytopathology. 1995;**85**:458-462

[51] Wishart J, Phillips MS, Blok VC. Ribosomal intergenic spacer: A PCR diagnostic for *Meloidogyne chitwoodi, M. fallax* and *M. hapla*. Phytopathology. 2002;**92**:884-892

[52] Zijlstra C, van Hoof R, Donkers-Venne D. A PCR test to detect the cereal root-knot nematode *Meloidogyne naasi*. European Journal of Plant Pathology. 2004;**110**:855-860

[53] Castagnone C, Abad P, Castagnone-Sereno P. Satellite DNA-based species-specific identification of single individuals of the pinewood nematode *Bursaphelenchus xylophilus* (Nematoda: Aphelenchoididae). European Journal of Plant Pathology. 2005;**112**:191-193

[54] François C, Castagnone C, Boonham N, Tomlinson J, Lawson R. Satellite DNA as a target for TaqMan real-time PCR detection of the pinewood nematode, *Bursaphelenchus xylophilus*. Molecular Plant Pathology. 2007;**8**:803-809

[55] Leal I, Green M, Allen E, Humble L, Rott M. Application of a real-time PCR method for the detection of pine wood nematode, *Bursaphelenchas xylophilus*, in wood samples from lodgepole pine. Nematology. 2007;**9**:351-362

[56] Jeszke A, Dobosz R, Obrępalska-Stęplowska A. A fast and sensitive method for the simultaneous identification of three important nematode species of the genus *Ditylenchus*. Pest Management Science. 2015;**71**(2):243-249

[57] Goto K, Sato E, Toyota K. A novel detection method for the soybean cyst nematode *Heterodera glycines* Ichinohe using soil compaction and real-time PCR. Japanese Journal of Nematology. 2009;**39**:1-7

[58] Amiri S, Subottin SA, Moens M. Identification of the beet cyst nematode *Heterodera schachtii* by PCR. European Journal of Plant Pathology. 2002;**108**:497-506

[59] Ye W. Development of prime time Real Time PCR for species identification of soybean cyst nematode (*Heterodera glycines* Ichinohe, 1952) in North Carolina. Journal of Nematology. 2012;**44**(3):284-290

[60] Sato E, Min YY, Shirakashi T, Wada S, Toyota K. Detection of the root-lesion nematode, *Pratylenchus penetrans* (Cobb), in a nematode community using real-time PCR. Japanese Journal of Nematology. 2017;**37**:87-92

[61] Adam MAM, Philips MS, Blok VC. Molecular diagnostic key for identification of single juveniles of seven common and economically important species of root-knot nematode (*Meloidogyne* spp.). Plant Pathology. 2007;**56**(1):190-197

[62] Floyd R, Abebe E, Papert A, Blaxter ML. Molecular barcodes for soil nematode identification. Molecular Ecology. 2002;**11**:839-850

[63] Chen Q, Robertson L, Jones JT, Blok VC, Phillips MS, Brown DJF. Capture of nematodes using antiserum and lectin-coated magnetized beads. Nematology. 2001;**3**:593-601

Chapter 3

Molecular Diagnostic Tools for Nematodes

Michalakis Christoforou, Michael Orford and
Dimitris Tsaltas

Additional information is available at the end of the chapter

http://dx.doi.org/10.5772/intechopen.69075

Abstract

The phylum of Nematoda is a species-rich taxonomic group in abundant numbers across a wide range of habitats, including plant and animal pathogens, as well as good environmental health indicators. Morphological observations are of low throughput and more importantly have problems with their discriminatory capacity, particularly at the species level. For these reasons, diagnostic tools are of paramount importance for all fields of human, animal and plant nematology as well as for environmental studies in water and soil. Accurate, fast and low-cost methodologies are required in order to identify and quantify the population of nematodes in samples from various sources. Scientists in basic research as well as in routine application fields need to have tools for resolving these identification obstacles. Their decisions can be human-, animal- or plant-health related, while many times legally committing. As a result, applicable and accredited methods are required and should be readily available in a common routine lab or in the field of battle or at border control agencies. This chapter aims to inform with the most current information on the available tools for nematode diagnostics, their positives and negatives and hints about the trends in the field and suggestions for those who would like to pursue further this field of biotechnology as researchers or simple users.

Keywords: nematode, detection, quantification, diagnostics, PCR, qPCR, DNA barcoding, Sequencing, NGS, MALDI-TOF

1. Introduction

Nematode identification is crucial for nematologists, diagnosticians and policy-makers. Due to the nematodes small size, life cycle and different habitats, scientists have been struggling to find morphological differences among species that would differentiate them. Nematode identification and differentiation can provide accurate decisions for the control of parasitic nematodes and the conservation of non-parasitic nematodes. Many misidentifications due to morphological errors resulted in huge economic impacts around the world. In the 1970s, plant parasitic nematode (PPN) control was based on the use of soil fumigants which made the species identification unnecessary whereas nowadays, the prohibition of those chemicals necessitates the accurate identification of species for the effective implementation of non-chemical management strategies [1].

A huge step towards nematode identification has been the use of biochemical and molecular diagnostic tools such as the enzyme-linked immunosorbent assay (ELISA) [2], isoelectric focusing (IEF) [3] and the polymerase chain reaction (PCR) [4]. The first two biochemical methods, ELISA and IEF, have received limited use as diagnostic tools due to appearance of the most effective, precise and fast PCR-based methods with the use of DNA which has provided solutions in several identification problems. The internal transcribed spacer (ITS) has proven to be a useful DNA region from which universal or species-specific primers are used in PCR reactions. The ITS regions are considered to be the most widely used for identification purposes by nematologists [5]. The use of PCR technology enables nematologists to diagnose nematode diseases rapidly and accurately. Furthermore, the use of PCR is adopted by the European and Mediterranean Plant Protection Organization (EPPO) and used in standardized protocols [6].

2. DNA extraction methods

Plenty of DNA extraction methods have been reported for DNA extraction, from single juveniles to a large number of juveniles, eggs or cysts. DNA extraction methods include commercial kits such as silica columns to bind DNA and switchable magnetic-based surface technology, Chelex® resin, phenol/chloroform and a worm lysis buffer (WLB). From all the methods mentioned above, the silica columns provide the highest quality DNA even from soil samples [7] and thus are widely used by many laboratories despite them being more than three times expensive than the others [8]. Phenol/chloroform is a method widely used before the emergence of commercial kits and although it is still a satisfactory method which provides pure and good-quality DNA template, it is avoided by researchers due toxic effects. Chelex® 100 is a chelating resin that uses ion exchange to bind transition metal ions. The resin is composed of styrene divinylbenzene copolymers containing paired iminodiacetate ions, which act a chelator for polyvalent metal ions. During the extraction process, the alkalinity of the solution and the act of boiling the solution break down the cells and allow the chelating groups to bind to the cellular components, thus protecting the DNA from degradation [9]. Chelex® resin and WLB are two inexpensive methods, rapid and easy to apply and will be presented in this chapter.

2.1. Chelex® resin protocol

1. Prepare 5–10% Chelex® resin solution using deionized water.

2. Boil the nematode (juveniles or cysts) at 95°C for 5 min in the 10% Chelex® resin solution.

3. Centrifuge at 20,000× for 1 min to separate the resin and cellular debris from the supernatant which contains the DNA template.

http://dx.doi.org/10.5772/intechopen.69075

2.2. Worm lysis buffer: single-worm DNA extraction

1. Prepare the WLB solution by mixing 50-mM KCl, 10-mM Tris, pH 8.2, 2.5-mM $MgCl_2$, 60-μg/ml proteinase K, 0.45% NP40 (Fisher Scientific), 0.45% Tween 20 (Sigma) and 0.01% gelatine [10].
2. Place the juvenile in 10 μL of WLB on a glass microscope slide.
3. Cut the nematode into two pieces using a sterile fine scalpel blade under a stereomicroscope.
4. Transfer the cut nematode using a pipette into a 0.2-ml centrifuge tube containing another 10 μL of WLB.
5. Centrifuge at 13,500 rp.m. for 2 min and then place at −80°C for 15 min.
6. Incubate the nematodes at 60°C for 1 h, followed by 95°C for 10 min to inactivate the proteinase K.
7. Freeze the DNA samples at −20 °C until ready for use.

2.3. Phenol/chloroform extraction/cleanup of genomic DNA

2.3.1. Digestion

1. Drop tissue pieces into liquid nitrogen to freeze.
2. Using a mortar and pestle, crush and grind the frozen tissue to make a powder.
3. Transfer to 50-ml tube and briefly spin to pack tissues to the bottom of tube.
4. Add TNES buffer (50-mM Tris-HCl, pH 7.5, 400-mM NaCl, 100-mM EDTA, pH 8.0 and 0.5% SDS-containing proteinase K (20 mg/ml) to bring volume to around 10 ml).
5. Incubate overnight at 50°C.
6. Adjust to 1.5-M NaCl (add an equal volume of 2.6 M NaCl).
7. Shake vigorously for 30 s.
8. Centrifuge 12,000× g for 5 min.
9. Decant the supernatant to a fresh tube and add an equal volume of ethanol.
10. Spool out the DNA and dissolve in 500 μl of water.

2.3.2. Extraction

1. Add an equal volume of phenol/chloroform/isoamyl alcohol to the DNA solution.
2. Vortex vigorously for 10 s and microcentrifuge for 15 s at room temperature.

3. Carefully remove the top (aqueous) phase containing the DNA and transfer to a new tube. If a white precipitate is present at the aqueous/organic interface, re-extract the organic phase and pool the aqueous phases.
4. Add 1/10 volume of 3-M sodium acetate, pH 5.2, to the solution of DNA. Mix by vortexing briefly.
5. Add 2–2.5 vol of ice cold 100% ethanol. Mix by vortexing and place in crushed dry ice for 5 min or longer.
6. Spin 20 min at 13,000× g in the microcentrifuge and remove the supernatant.
7. Add 1 ml of room temperature 70% ethanol. Invert the tube several times and microcentrifuge for 5 min at 13,000× g.
8. Remove the supernatant. Allow to air dry for 15 min.
9. Re-suspend DNA pellet in 100 μl of ultra-pure water or TE buffer.

3. PCR-based methods

PCR-based methods involve the extraction of DNA from single or numerous juveniles, nematocysts or complex soil samples. The PCR-based molecular diagnostic tools used for nematode identification and quantification are restriction fragment length polymorphisms (RFLPs), ribosomal DNA (rDNA) PCR, mitochondrial DNA amplification, microsatellite DNA fragment analysis, real-time PCR, microarrays, sequence-characterized amplified regions (SCARs) and next-generation sequencing (NGS).

3.1. Restriction fragment length polymorphisms

In Ref. [11], Curran et al. differentiated the Meloidogyne population on the level of race and strains by using total genome analysis from washed eggs. The egg DNA was purified and digested with *Eco*RI and electrophoresed in an agarose gel and visualized [11]. Due to the large number of specimens and thus the high amount of DNA needed for RFLPs analysis, the technique was improved in the early 1990s with the use DNA hybridization [12, 13] and finally PCR [4]. The combination of amplification and digestion (PCR-RFLP) of a single DNA strand has been found useful for DNA comparisons among individual nematodes [5]. Various PCR products during restriction endonuclease digestion lead to differences in fragment length within the restriction site yielding different RFLP profiles. To obtain a desirable result, different digestive enzymes participate. Nonetheless, the digestive enzymes used in RFLP do not separate all species within a genus, an issue that will be overcome with the use of species-specific primers. The specificity of RFLP could be used for the examination of a broad range of isolates from different sites around the world and thus confirm the general applicability of the RFLP method [14]. Nevertheless, as a diagnostic tool, PCR-RFLP could eliminate much of the ambiguity involved in morphological identification of nematode specimens since differences in RFLP can be presented as the existence of differences in restriction sites in the ITS sequence (**Figure 1**) [15, 16]. Nowadays, PCR-RFLP is still used when species-specific primers are absent.

3.2. Ribosomal DNA polymerase chain reaction (rDNA-PCR)

PCR brought the evolution in molecular diagnostics of nematodes since the early 1990s. Primers were designed to produce large DNA products from which species-specific primers were then designed for producing unique products of each species. By the late 1990s, species-specific primers were designed for quarantine species such as *Globodera pallida* and *Globodera rostochiensis* [17, 18]. Nematode PCR products were derived from the 18S, 28S, 5,8S coding genes and the ITS regions. The ITS region is considered a variable area of DNA that has been repeatedly examined for molecular differences among species. In 1996, Mulholland et al. [19] presented a multiplex PCR technique based on the use of species-specific primers, able to identify potato cyst nematodes (PCN) at the species level and without the use of restriction endonuclease digestion [19].

The PCR method requires DNA extracted from specimens, two pairs of 12–24-bp oligonucleotides named primers, which are complimentary to the 3′end of each strand in a specific binding site of the DNA region that will be amplified, a DNA polymerase (*Taq* DNA polymerase), four deoxynucleotides (dATP, dCTP, dGTP and dTTP) and a buffer-containing $MgCl_2$. The steps of the PCR method contain the activation of the Taq DNA polymerase (usually above 90°C), the denaturation of the DNA chain into two separated strands (usually above 90°C), the annealing of the primers (between 45 and 65°C) and the extension of the new strands, which involves the attachment of the Taq enzyme on the primers 3′end and the moving of the enzyme downstream along the DNA template, incorporating the free dNTPs on the new strand. The extension process is usually done at 72°C. PCR method usually uses around 35–40

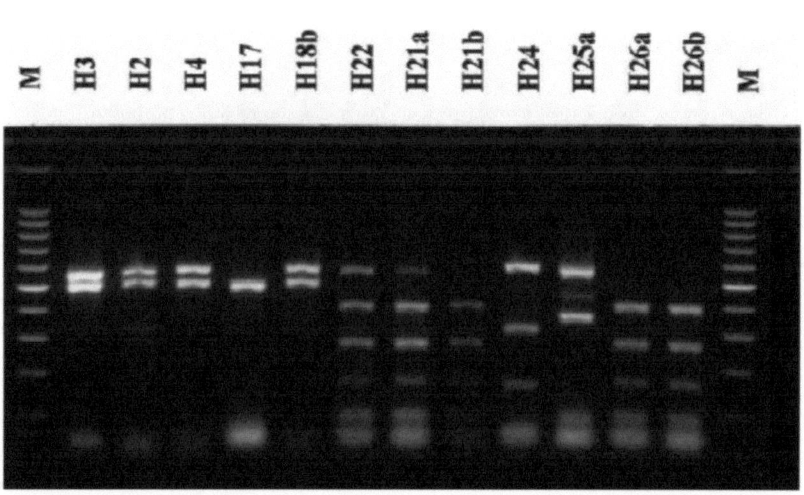

Figure 1. Restriction fragments of amplified ITS regions of cyst-forming nematodes digested by *Tru*9I. M: 100 bp ladder and H: Heterodera species [15].

cycles in a PCR thermocycler. The PCR product is mixed with a fluorescent dye and then transferred into separated wells of agarose gel, with the first well having a DNA ladder used as molecular weight marker. The loaded agarose gel is placed in a tray with buffer (the same buffer with which the gel was prepared) and plugged with electrodes (− electrode in the wells side and + electrode in the other site of the tray) at 100 volts. The higher the voltage, the faster the DNA moves but the heat increases and thus decreases resolution. Agarose gel is then visualized in UV light and photographed. Fleming *et al.* [20], used the PCR method for diagnosing and estimating population levels of PCN. They demonstrated a correlation between the number of viable juveniles hatched from a cyst with the amount of DNA that could be extracted from them in a quantitative manner [20]. A multiplex PCR was presented by Bulman and Marshal, (**Figure 2**), when species-specific primers were used and combined with mixed populations of PCNs [17]. A few years later, the PCR method was named conventional PCR (CoPCR) due the appearance of quantitative real-time PCR (qPCR) [21].

3.3. Real-time PCR

While conventional PCR was used worldwide for identification purposes, there was a need for more rapid, sensitive and cost-efficient method for identifying nematodes. As the genome analysis was heading deeper and deeper, more and more sequence data became available which made nematode identification and species discrimination more rapid and accurate [22]. Real-time PCR provides simultaneous amplification of the DNA target sequence and direct analysis of the PCR products by incorporating fluorescent probes or dyes into the reaction mix and thus the need for gel electrophoresis is avoided [23]. In real-time PCR, the fluorescent molecule (probe or dye) reports the amount of DNA as it is multiplied in each cycle as the fluorescent signal increases proportionally. The two types of fluorescent molecules used in real-time PCR bind on DNA as DNA-binding dyes or fluorescently labelled specific primers

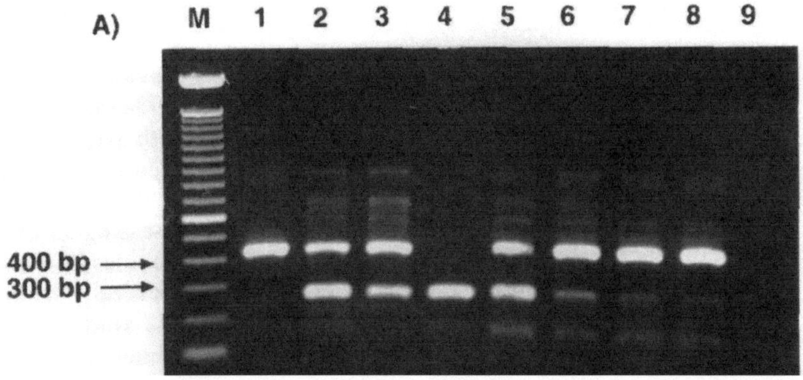

Figure 2. Polymerase chain reaction (PCR) differentiation of the potato cyst nematode (PCN) species, *Globodera rostochiensis* and *Globodera pallida*, with various concentrations of DNA. A: multiplex PCR with primers Plp4, Plr3 and ITS% upon DNA from Ro1 Lincoln and Pa2/3 Lincoln. M: ladder, Lane 1, Ro1 1:20 H_2O, Lane 2, Ro1 1:20 Pa2/3, Lane 3, Ro1 1:1 Pa2/3 (1:20 H_2O each), Lane 4, Pa2/3 1:20 H_2O, Lane 5, Ro1 10:1 Pa2/3, Lane 6, Ro1 20:1 Pa2/3, Lane 7, Ro1 50:1 Pa2/3, Lane 8, Ro1 100:1 Pa2/3, Lane 9, no DNA control [17].

or probes and specialized thermal cyclers detect, monitor and measure the fluorescence which reflects the amount of the amplified products in each cycle, in real time.

Quantitative real-time PCR is used for the detection and quantification of DNA present in a sample which is reflected by the number of nematodes present in the sample. For the quantification of nematodes using qPCR, a standard curve is needed (**Figure 3**) [24]. Standard curves are constructed by plotting the Ct values against the logarithm of the DNA amount isolated from different amounts of nematode eggs and juveniles. The amplification efficiency (*E*) is calculated from the slope of the standard curve using the following formula $E = 10^{[-1/\text{slope}]} - 1$ [25]. qPCR is used for the quantitative detection, species identification and discrimination in plant and in veterinary parasitic nematodes [8, 23, 24, 26–30].

Although quantification of nematodes was a step forward for estimating population levels of parasitic nematodes in a sample, the stability of DNA from dead specimens in samples especially those extracted from cysts appears to be an obstacle [26]. In the case of PCN, it is very common for dead juveniles to be present within a cyst (in-egg mortality) [31] and their DNA intact, while in soil, dead juveniles' DNA can be degraded in a short time. The DNA of *Phasmarhabditis hermaphrodita* was degraded in unpasteurized soil within 6 days as the dead juveniles were in direct contact to soil microflora [7]. Christoforou et al. [24] reported the detection and amplification of nematodes DNA in a 34-year-old cyst stored at room temperature using PCR (**Figure 4**) and qPCR with Taqman probes.

Although the use of DNA appears to be the best approach for live/dead specimen differentiation, its stability outside cell membranes allows the amplification of outbound DNA from dead cells as well, thus introducing inaccuracies in live nematode quantification. Recently, a

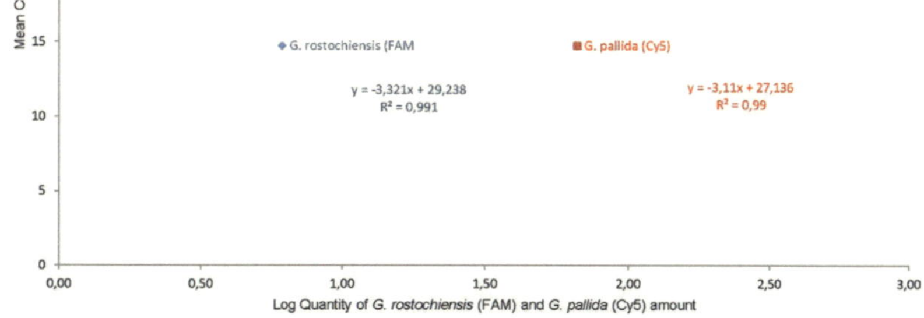

Figure 3. PMA-qPCR method for the detection and quantification of viable potato cyst nematodes. A: standard curves generated by duplex real-time PCR using DNA isolated from standard PCN solutions containing 1, 5, 25, 125 and 625 live eggs or juveniles (J2), respectively. The mean Ct values corresponding to the PCR cycle number are plotted against the logarithmic quantity of nematodes DNA used in triplicate as standards. The error bars represent standard deviations of three samples [24].

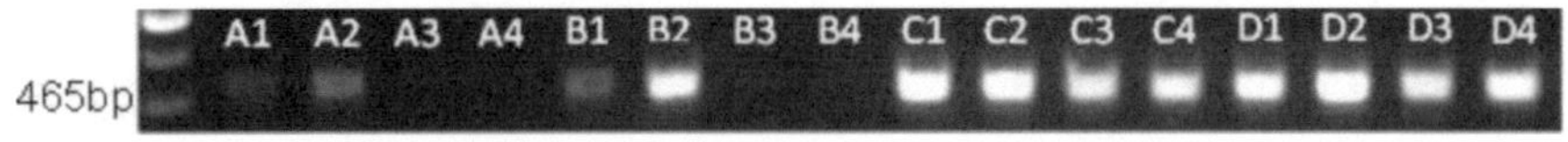

Figure 4. PCR-amplified products at 465 bp of genomic DNA from non-PMA and PMA-treated cysts (A1–A4: 1976, A1 and A2 non-PMA and A3 and A4 PMA; B1–B4: 1990, B1 and B2 non-PMA and B3 and B4 PMA; C1–C4: 2007, C1 and C2 non-PMA and C3 and C4 PMA; D1–D4: 2010, D1 and D2 non-PMA and D3 and D4 PMA) [24].

new chemical dye propidium monoazide (PMA) has been used for selective detection of viable bacteria, fungi and nematodes, in combination with qPCR [24, 32–34]. PMA is a photoreactive DNA-intercalating dye which renders exposed DNA of dead cells, is unable to amplify and thus, only DNA from viable/intact cells is PCR amplified and detected. Christoforou *et. al.* [24], presented a qualitative estimation of viable PCN inocula using species-specific primers and Taqman probes designed by Papayiannis *et al.* [8], in a PMA-qPCR method which was developed for the two PCN species. The PMA-qPCR method successfully discriminates dead from living specimens in heat-treated samples as also the eggs from old and newly formed cysts.

qPCR method proves to be very useful for routine identification and discrimination of nematode species from field samples. The optimization of the qPCR and DNA extraction methods is essential for the specificity, sensitivity and accuracy of the procedure. Madani *et al.* [26], described a real-time PCR method using SYBR green-I dye with melting curve analysis for the detection and quantification of PCN species and mentioned the dependence of nematode quantification on the efficacy of DNA-extraction methods. Papayiannis *et al.* [8], evaluated five DNA extraction methods (silica columns, magnetic-based surface, Chelex resin, chloroform-based and disruption in TE) and compared them for their preparation time, cost and technical difficulty as well as the limit of detection between PCR and qPCR assays for all extraction methods. Another important factor for an accurate qPCR assay is the primers' specificity and the limitations in detecting nematodes when species are mixed in a sample. When three plant parasitic nematodes (PPNs), *Meloidogyne javanica, Pratylenchus zeae* and *Xiphinema elongatum,* were tested for identification and quantification in a mixture of species and primers, competition between the DNA of *M. javanica* with *P. zeae* and *X. elongatum* was found [27].

4. Microarrays

Microarrays show high potential for discriminating nematodes in multi-complex samples since many targets can be identified simultaneously due to the specificity of the microarray method to detect unique sequences for each target species [35, 36]. Microarrays are composed of complementary DNAs (cDNAs) that can be detected due to a fluorescence bind on the cDNA, on microscope slides or silicon chips, which contain specific synthesized known DNA after hybridization of the cDNA. Ahmed et al. [36] mentioned the potential of using the microarrays to identify gastrointestinal nematodes. Besides the high prospective of microarrays as diagnostic tools for identifying nematodes, it still has not been achievable. The high cost, the amplification of unknown sequences in mixed samples and the better hybridization of mismatched targets rather than the perfectly matched targets lead to the limited use of the microarray method as a diagnostic tool for nematodes [35].

5. DNA sequencing

DNA sequencing or DNA barcoding is referred to many nematode-related publications and has been the main driving force in studies, and as availability of instrumentation increases while cost is constantly reduced, it is apparent that it will be the dominating approach. The Sanger method or NGS approaches accumulate a substantial amount of genetic data with sufficient, if not to say overwhelming, information on sequence divergence, which may be often characterized as erroneous due to sample or analysis limitations.

For diagnostic purposes, most studies have targeted two main genomic regions for sequence divergence. These regions are the nuclear ribosomal RNA genes and their transcribed and untranscribed spacers and the mitochondrial cytochrome oxidase I (COI) gene. These regions are highly conserved but sufficiently divergent and occur in multiple copies in the genome, thus made easily amplifiable by PCR. A key element of this approach is the use of standardized markers and a relatively standardized experimental approach not introducing significant subjectiveness. On the other hand, this methodology builds taxonomic reference libraries where all submitted sequences from different organisms can be compared. As a result, unidentified organisms can be determined according to the level of DNA homology [37]. Results can be acquired in as fast as 8–12 h, making the method competent to be used in control of pest movement within trade activities and border control [38]. rDNA genes are preferred over COI gene in most studies due to the availability of sequences and the level of conservation in order to design universal primers even though COI is capable of discriminating between species at a better level. Porazinska et al. [39] had shown that the use of SSU and LSU genes together improves resolution.

With the development of NGS approaches, similarly to metagenomics, a term that has been used solely for microorganisms, DNA metabarcoding, is rapidly evolving. Bulk DNA deriving from environmental samples (water, soil) but same approach can be applied elsewhere (i.e. infected plant tissues, animal gut, blood samples), can uncover the entire hidden microcosm [37]. This approach can be used both for ecology studies, including soil quality and health, and for plant/animal diagnostics.

Limitations of high-throughput DNA barcoding still exist and are mainly the following: (1) Efficiency of DNA recovery is an issue but experimentation and protocol development studies will soon address this, (2) identification of a suitable marker to provide good taxonomic coverage and species resolution and (3) formation of chimeras (artefacts of PCR when an incompletely extended DNA fragment from one cycle anneals to a template of an unrelated taxon and gets copied to completion in subsequent cycles). Bioinformatic tools are trained to identify and discard such sequences.

The second limitation referred to above can be indirectly resolved by taking advantage of the high throughput of NGS technology, where multiple genes can be simultaneously sequenced and analysed with relatively low cost. In our times, genetic information will be easily acquired and our main technical obstacle is the vastness of information in genetic repositories of sequences, that storage and computing capacities require constant upgrade to convey biological and taxonomic meanings to scientists.

It is worth referring the most recent achievement of DNA sequencing, using third-generation sequencing technology and providing whole genome analysis that has used the portable device MinION. Tyson et al. [40] have reported performing the whole genome and assembly of a *Caenorhabditis elegans* genome with complex genomic arrangements. Two astonishing elements of this study are the USB type and sized instrument of MinION and the long reads that the technology offers. This second attribute improves immensely the NGS technology for de novo sequencing of complex genomes, in part due to repeat regions that nematodes as metazoans have in common. The flowcell of MinION is currently able to provide 5–10 Gb of sequence, which is a sufficient performance for a 100-Mb genome of a nematode with long reads for an unambiguous assembly of the chromosome.

6. Other methods

A variety of biochemical methods have been used in the past for nematode identification. They relied mainly on protein analysis using isoelectric focusing, two-dimensional electrophoresis and serological techniques using monoclonal or polyclonal antibodies. None of these techniques reached an application level, and research has been seized. Recently, the use of analytical instrumentation for protein analysis has acquired the attention of the research and application scientific community. MALDI-TOF mass spectrometry is a method that can be used for microorganism's identification [41] and has been reported by Pepera et al. [42] for nematodes as well with very good results. The authors discriminated up to a race level for *Ditylenchus dipsaci*. Although in microorganisms the ribosomal proteins seem to be the prominent identification/fingerprinting molecules, in this report [42], an array of other proteins of housekeeping importance were analysed and sequenced (LC MS/MS). The discriminatory differences found on proteomic approaches such as the aforementioned can more easily contribute and lead to the identification of pathogenicity factors important for development of new disease management strategies, through resistant plant cultivars. Conclusively, MALDI-TOF technology beside the instrumentation cost (in 2017, prices are about 150–200 K euros) is a robust technique, with very low cost per sample preparation and analysis (1-h for sample preparation and 3 min for analysis). Similar to microbial proteomic instrumentation, commercially available databases (Bruker MALDI Biotyper, Biomerieux VITEK MS) can be developed for nematode identification.

7. Conclusions

Molecular diagnostics are used as tools for the identification of parasitic and free-living nematodes since the early 1990s. Currently, most of the veterinary and plant protection laboratories use molecular tools for the identification, discrimination and quantification of important parasitic nematodes for common everyday diagnostic activities. From all the molecular tools and methods mentioned in the literature and in this review, only few are used in routine protocols. These selected ones are highly correlated with the reliability, the time and cost effectiveness as well as the expertise necessary for applying the methods.

From the methods reviewed in this chapter, real-time PCR is currently the fastest, most-sensitive and accurate method. Taqman PCR assay could detect, identify and quantify nematodes, reaching 100% accuracy. Real-time PCR methodologies can be of use in field applications with the use of a mobile qPCR instrument that is able to operate in field conditions along with easy-to-perform kits like DNA extraction and PCR reaction chemistries. For more analytical protocols and methodologies, DNA barcoding is fast progressing as DNA sequencing tools develop. However, we need to inform our readers that DNA barcoding based on NGS technologies and proteomic analysis based on mass spectrometry will soon dominate the market and offer low-budget, kit-type applications even for mobile diagnostic laboratories.

Author details

Michalakis Christoforou, Michael Orford and Dimitris Tsaltas*

*Address all correspondence to: dimitris.tsaltas@cut.ac.cy

Department of Agricultural Sciences, Biotechnology and Food Science, Cyprus University of Technology, Limassol, Republic of Cyprus

References

[1] Hyman BC. Molecular diagnosis of Meloidogyne species. Journal of Nematology. 1990; **22**:24-30

[2] Sutanto I, Maizels RM, Denham DA. Surface antigens of a filarial nematode: Analysis of adult *Brugia pahangi* surface components and their use in monoclonal antibody production. Molecular and Biochemical Parasitology. 1985;**15**:203-210

[3] Lawson EC, Carter GE, Lewis SA. Application of isoelectric focusing to the taxonomic identification of Meloidogyne spp. Journal of Nematology. 1984;**16**:91-96

[4] Harris TS, Sandall LJ, Powers TO. Identification of single *Meloidogyne juveniles* by polymerase chain reaction amplification of mitochondrial DNA. Journal of Nematology. 1990;**22**:518-524

[5] Powers TO, Todd TC, Burnell AM, Murray PC, Fleming CC, Szalanski AL, et al. The rDNA internal transcribed spacer region as a taxonomic marker for nematodes. Journal of Nematology. 1997;**29**:441-450

[6] EPPO b. PM 7/4 (3) *Bursaphelenchus xylophilus*. Wiley Online Library Website 2013;**43**: 105-118

[7] MacMillan K, Blok V, Young I, Crawford J, Wilson MJ. Quantification of the slug parasitic nematode *Phasmarhabditis hermaphrodita* from soil samples using real time qPCR. International Journal of Parasitology. 2006;**36**(14):1453-1461

[8] Papayiannis LC, Christoforou M, Markou Y, Tsaltas D. Molecular typing of cyst-forming nematodes *Globodera pallida* and *G. rostochiensis*, using real-time PCR and evaluation of five methods for template preparation. Journal of Phytopathology. 2013;161:459-469

[9] Bio-Rad L. Chelex®-100 and Chelex®-20 Chelating Ion Exchange Resin Instruction Manual. Bio-Rad Laboratories, 2000 Alfred Nobel Dr., Hercules, CA 94547 LIT200 Rev B

[10] Castagnone-Sereno P, Esparrago G, Abad P, Leroy F, Bongiovanni M. Satellite DNA as a target for PCR-specific detection of the plant-parasitic nematode *Meloidogyne hapla*. Current Genetics. 1995;**28**(6):566-570

[11] Curran J, McClure MA, Webster JM. Genotypic differentiation of Meloidogyne populations by detection of restriction fragment length difference in total DNA. Journal of Nematology. 1986;**18**(1):83-86

[12] Schnick D, Rumpenhorst H, Burgermeister W. Differentiation of closely related *Globodera pallida* (stone) populations by means of DNA restriction fragment length polymorphisms (RFLPs). Journal of Phytopathology. 1990;**130**:127-136

[13] Dalmasso A. Phylogenetic relationships between amphimictic and parthenogenetic nematodes of the genus Meloidogyne as inferred from repetitive DNA analysis. Heredity. 1993;**70**:195-204

[14] Powers TO, Harris TS. A polymerase chain reaction method for identification of five major Meloidogyne species. Journal of Nematology. 1993;**25**:1-6

[15] Subbotin SA, Waeyenberge L, Moens M. Identification of cyst forming nematodes of the genus Heterodera (Nematoda: Heteroderidae) based on the ribosomal DNA-RFLP. Nematology. 2000;**2**:153-164

[16] Powers TO, Szalanski AL, Mullin PG, Harris TS, Bertozzi T, Griesbach JA. Identification of seed gall nematodes of agronomic and regulatory concern with PCR-RFLP of ITS1. Journal of Nematology. 2001;**33**:191-194

[17] Bulman S, Marshall J. Differentiation of Australasian potato cyst nematode (PCN) populations using the polymerase chain reaction (PCR). New Zealand Journal of Crop and Horticultural Science. 1997;**25**(2):123-129

[18] Fullaondo A, Barrena E, Viribay M, Barrena I, Salazar A, Ritter E. Identification of potato cyst nematode species *Globodera rostochiensis* and *G. pallida* by PCR using specific primer combinations. Nematology. 1999;**1**(2):157-163

[19] Mulholland V, Carde L, O'Donnell K, Fleming CC, Powers T. Diagnostics in crop production. BCPC Symposium Proceedings. 1996;**65**:247-256

[20] Fleming CC, Turner SJ, Powers TO, Szalansky AL. Diagnostics of cyst nematodes: Use of the polymerase chain reaction to determine species and estimate population levels. Aspects of Applied Biology. 1998;**52**:375-382

[21] Bates JA, Taylor EJA, Gans PT, Thomas JE, Bates JA. Determination of relative proportions of Globodera species in mixed populations of potato cyst nematodes using PCR product melting peak analysis. Molecular Plant Pathology. 2002;**3**:153-161

[22] Schaad NW, Frederick RD. Real-time PCR and its application for rapid plant disease diagnostics. Canadian Journal of Plant Pathology. 2002;**24**(3):250-258

[23] Zarlenga DS, Higgins J. PCR as a diagnostic and quantitative technique in veterinary parasitology. Veterinary Parasitology. 2001;**101**(3):215-230

[24] Christoforou M, Pantelides I, Kanetis L, Ioannou N, Tsaltas D. Rapid detection and quantification of viable potato cyst nematodes using qPCR in combination with propidium monoazide. Plant Pathology. 2014;**63**(5):1185-1192

[25] Pfaffl M. A new mathematical model for relative quantification in real-time RT-PCR. Nucleic Acids Research 2001;**29**:45

[26] Madani M, Subbotin SA, Moens M. Quantitative detection of the potato cyst nematode, *Globodera pallida*, and the beet cyst nematode, *Heterodera schachtii*, using real-time PCR with SYBR green I dye. Molecular and Cellular Probes. 2005;**19**(2):81-86

[27] Berry SD, Fargette M, Spaull VW, Morand S, Cadet P. Detection and quantification of root-knot nematode (*Meloidogyne javanica*), lesion nematode (*Pratylenchus zeae*) and dagger nematode (*Xiphinema elongatum*) parasites of sugarcane using real-time PCR. Molecular and Cellular Probes. 2008;**22**(3):168-176

[28] Nowaczyk K, Dobosz R, Kornobis S, Obrepalska-Steplowska A. TaqMan real-time PCR-based approach for differentiation between *Globodera rostochiensis* (golden nematode) and *Globodera artemisiae* species. Parasitology Research. 2008;**103**(3):577-581

[29] Madani M, Ward LJ, De Boer SH. Multiplex real-time polymerase chain reaction for identifying potato cyst nematodes, *Globodera pallida* and *Globodera rostochiensis*, and the tobacco cyst nematode, *Globodera tabacum*. Canadian Journal of Plant Pathology. 2008;**30**(4):554-564

[30] Nakhla KM, Owens KJ, Wei WLG, Skantar AM, Levy L. Multiplex real-time PCR assays for the identification of the potato cyst and tobacco cyst nematodes. Pest Management Science. 2010;**8**:959-965

[31] Devine KJ, Byrne J, Jones PW. In vitro studies on the relative availability and mobility in soil of natural hatching factors for the potato cyst nematodes, *Globodera rostochiensis* and *G. pallida*. Nematology. 2001;**3**(1):75-83

[32] Nocker A, Sossa KE, Camper AK. Molecular monitoring of disinfection efficacy using propidium monoazide in combination with quantitative PCR. Journal of Microbiological Methods. 2007;**70**(2):252-260

[33] Bae S, Wuertz S. Discrimination of viable and dead fecal Bacteroidales bacteria by quantitative PCR with propidium monoazide. Applied and Environmental Microbiology. 2009;**75**(9):2940-2944

[34] Vesper S, McKinstry C, Hartmann C, Neace M, Yoder S, Vesper A. Quantifying fungal viability in air and water samples using quantitative PCR after treatment with propidium monoazide (PMA). Journal of Microbiological Methods. 2008;**72**:180-184

[35] Blok VC, Powers TO. Biochemical and molecular identification. In: Root-Knot Nematodes. 2009, CABI, UK pp. 98-118

[36] Ahmed M, Singh M, Bera A, Bandyopadhyay S, Bhattacharya D. Molecular basis for identification of species/isolates of gastrointestinal nematode parasites. Asian Pacific Journal of Tropical Medicine. 2011;**4**(8):589-593

[37] Taberlet P, Coissac E, Pompanon F, Brochmann C, Willerslev E. Towards next-generation biodiversity assessment using DNA metabarcoding. Molecular Ecology. 2012;**21**: 2045-2050

[38] Powers T. Nematode molecular diagnostics: From bands to barcodes. Annual Review of Phytopathology. 2004;**42**:367-383

[39] Porazinska D, Giblin-Davis R, Faller L, Farmerie W, Kanzaki N, Morris K, et al. Evaluating high-throughput sequencing as a method for metagenomic analysis of nematode diversity. Molecular Ecology. 2009;**9**:1439-1450

[40] Tyson JR, O'Neil NJ, Jain M, Olsen HE, Hieter P, Snutch TP. Whole genome sequencing and assembly of a *Caenorhabditis elegans* genome with complex genomic rearrangements using the MinION sequencing device. bioRxiv. 2017. DOI: 10.1101/099143

[41] Singhal N, Kumar M, Kanaujia PK, Virdi JS. MALDI-TOF mass spectrometry: An emerging technology for microbial identification and diagnosis. Frontiers in Microbiology. 2015;**6**:791

[42] Perera MR, Taylor SP, Vanstone VA, Jones MG. Protein biomarkers to distinguish oat and lucerne races of the stem nematode, *Ditylenchus dipsaci,* with quarantine significance for Western Australia. Nematology. 2009;**11**(4):555-563

Section 2

Control of Nematodes

Chapter 4

Searching for Better Methodologies for Successful Control of Termites Using Entomopathogenic Nematodes

Hugues Baïmey, Lionel Zadji, Léonard Afouda,
André Fanou, Régina Kotchofa and
Wilfrieda Decraemer

Additional information is available at the end of the chapter

http://dx.doi.org/10.5772/intechopen.69861

Abstract

Termites are social insects reported from many countries of the world. Some species of them are known to be beneficial to man, whereas some others cause substantial losses (billions of US dollars annually) of properties and amenities. Various preventive and remedial methods are used to control undesirable termite species. The current review paper gives an overview of beneficial and detrimental activities of termites. Methods of control of undesirable species of termites are given and their advantages and disadvantages are discussed. We emphasized on the use of entomopathogenic nematodes (EPNs) as effective, environmentally safe and sustainable biological control method against termites. Species of EPNs recovered in Africa are documented. Some techniques used to collect termites and to maintain them for experiments and also to propagate, to formulate, to store, and to check for the quality of EPNs for application in the laboratory and in the field are also discussed. The environmental factors affecting the potential of EPNs to control termites are discussed. The information provided in this chapter will help researchers to enhance their skills of the use of EPNs against termites by selecting from the methodologies described here the best ones to adapt to particular experimental conditions, especially in African soil conditions.

Keywords: termites, entomopathogenic nematodes, biological control, methodology, Africa

1. Introduction

Termites belong to the order Isoptera [1] and include more than 3500 species described in the world [2]. Some of them play beneficial roles to man [3, 4], but some cause to him significant economic losses [5]. In both cases, there are different termites considering their habitats and caste type. In recent years, there has been a large increase in the scientific literature concerning termites [6]. The control of species of termites with detrimental effects relies mainly on soil chemical termiticide applications, especially in African countries. But despite this reliance on chemical termiticides, termite control strategies need to conform to higher environmental standards [7]. In this regard, several research projects focus their activities on biological control methods which are environmentally safe. Among these methods is the use of entomopathogenic nematodes (EPNs). These nematodes have a worldwide distribution [8]. Apart from being environmentally safe, the use of EPN in pest control in general, and in termite control in particular, is rapid, sustainable, and cost effective. For the use of EPNs to control termites, different research methodologies are considered. But the results of these researches are sometimes controversial. This is related to the origin and biology of the species of the nematodes, to the type of termites, but also to the environment where the nematodes have been applied. Usually, newly described EPN species are first tested under laboratory conditions before best isolated are selected and tested under field conditions. Even under those conditions, methodologies used to evaluate the performance of the nematodes vary with researchers [9], leading to different results. The current review paper gives information on termites with focus on those with detrimental effects to man. It also discusses several methodologies commonly used to study the characteristics and also the performance of EPNs in the control of termites.

2. Termites

2.1. Classification and distribution of termites

Like ants, wasps, and bees, termites are social insects. They constitute 10% of all animal biomass in the tropics. Baker and Marchosky [10] divided termites into three general categories based on their habitat: dampwood, drywood, and subterranean termites. A typical termite colony contains larvae, nymphs, workers, soldiers, and reproductives, each type having its specific role inside the nest. Termites are grouped into seven families and 15 subfamilies [11], 281 genera [12], and over 3500 species identified worldwide [13]. Africa has the richest intercontinental diversity of termites with over 70% of all the identified species [14]. The family Termitidae alone comprises more than 664 African species grouped in four subfamilies: Apicotermitinae with 70 species [15], Termitinae with 272 species [16], Macrotermitinae with 165 African fungus-growing termites [17], and Nasutitermitinae with 56 species [18]. The total number of species of termites in the four subfamilies may surpass 90% of the world's known termite species [14]. These authors reported species richness and diversity (see below the formulas for their calculation) as a result of the friendly climatic conditions in Africa, and that, dry climate is a factor contributing for low numbers of termite species in some regions of the world. For example, termite species diversity is lower in Northern Africa compared to Eastern, Western, and Southern regions of the continent [14]. Kemabonta et al. [19] also reported that termites are prominent in both tropical and subtropical ecosystems, but highest diversity is observed in tropical forests where they build very complex communities [16]. In recent years, there has been a large increase in the scientific literature concerning termites [6]. The different researches done on termites indicated their beneficial activities as well as detrimental effects to man.

Formulas are used to calculate termite species richness and diversity according to Ref. [19].

Termite species richness is calculated using the Shannon-Wiener diversity Index (H') as follows:

$H' = -\Sigma\ (P_i \ln P_i)$, where P_i is the proportion of individuals found in the ith species, while ln is the natural logarithm.

Termite diversity D is calculated using the Simpson index as $D = \sum_{i=1}^{S}(-1)/N(N-1)$, where n_i is the number of individuals in the ith species, while N is the total number of entities in the dataset.

2.2. Beneficial activities of termites

Termites play a major role in peoples' lives, in physical as well as spiritual aspects [20]. Reis de Figueirêdo et al. [21] cataloged 43 species of termites, belonging to four families used in human diet and/or in livestock feeding and nine species used as a therapeutic resource. These authors registered termite use in 29 countries over three countries: Africa (19), America (5), and Asia (5). Authors of Refs. [4, 5] reported that termites are of highly nutritive value. Their soil is often eaten by pregnant women in Africa [20]. Termites also play a role as oracle, in superstitious beliefs, art, and literature [20]. Their mounds are often associated with the spiritual world, especially containing the spirits of ancestors. In agriculture, termites produce organic matter from dead wood and woody tissues of plants, thereby restore organic matter to the soil and to air, serve as ecological indicators [22]. They play significant role in subsistence agriculture as their mounds, with nutrient enriched soils, are incorporated into traditional cropping systems. Termite mound materials are also made hard and used to make roads, tennis court, and bricks used in buildings and are also source of pottery clay [23]. In this book chapter, we will focus on termites as pests and their control.

2.3. Detrimental activities of termites

More than 300 species of termites are known to be of economic importance [5] causing billions of dollars in damage worldwide. Since their food supply is mainly wood and woody tissues of plants, they feed on anything containing cellulose component including crop residues, mulches, and humus. They cause damage to agricultural crops such as cash crops and food crops [2], timbers in buildings, fences, clothes, books [24], removal of plant covers exposing soil surface to erosive forces [25]. They cause economic losses by directly injuring and destroying both living and dead vegetation and can damage right from sowing the crops till harvest [26].

Baker and Marchosky [10] reported drywood and subterranean termites as the most significant and costly termite pests. They feed on a wide range of living, dead, or decaying plant material [16, 27], including the consumption and turnover of large volumes of soil rich in organic matter and fungi. These feeding habits make termites important ecosystem engineers, which over long periods of time can modify the physical properties of soil such as texture, water infiltration rates, and nutrient content [28]. They are among the most important insect pests in forests, and many destructive species live in the soil. For example, the forest termite *Coptotermes acinaciformis* causes more than 92% of total loss to Virgin *Eucalyptus pilularis*. In 2011, wood-eating termites consumed more than $220,000 worth of Indian rupee notes [29].

In West Africa, several species of termites, including *Macrotermes bellicosus, Macrotermes natalensis, Coptotermes sjostedti*, and *Pseudocanthotermes militaris*, have been reported as general pests of living trees. The establishment of eucalyptus is limited by two termite species, i.e., *Ancistrotermes cavithorax* and *Amitermes evincifer* in drier areas of Ghana. In this country, termite attack of living trees is a potentially important problem facing the use of exotic forest species. In Nigeria, termite pest species of the genus *Macrotermes* are the most destructive to plants causing 5–18% yield losses [3]. Ten species of termites were found associated with citrus orchards in Benin: *Amitermes guineensis, Ancistrotermes crucifer, Angulitermes truncates, Coptotermes intermedius, Cubitermes* sp., *M. bellicosus, Microcerotermes progrediens, Pericapritermes* sp., *Trinervitermes occidentalis*, and *Trinervitermes trinervius* [30]. Among these, *M. bellicosus*, a fungus-growing termite, is the most important species that undermines citrus production and *T. occidentalis*, a grass-feeder termite, the most important to maize, cassava, groundnut, and bean grown under citrus canopies [31]. Abe et al. [2] also reported that the most troublesome termites in agriculture are the fungus-growing termites. In the absence of crop residues, mulches, and humus, these termites eat live plant material as groundnuts, millets, and maize. *Odontotermes erraticus, Macrotermes sibhyalinus, Amitermes evuncifer, Psammotermes hybostoma*, and *Microtermes lepidus* with a wide predominance of the *O. erraticus* were found ravaging cassava in Tivaouane, Senegal [32]. In South Africa, *Coptotermes* spp., *Cryptotermes* spp., and *Neotermes* spp. were observed undermining crop productivity [33]. But since termites make openings to the outside, farmers are aware of their presence only at an advanced stage of their invasion [34]. In regard of all this, the menace of termite activities is enormous. It is then important to bring these activities to a manageable level. For experimental purposes, termites are collected and used immediately or maintained for days before use.

2.4. Termite collection and maintenance

Termites are cryptic social insects. If some of them live in galleries made on the surface of wood products (examples of plant stems and trunks), some others live deep in the soil or inside wood products. Methods for collecting them will therefore depend on their habitat structures. Wang et al. [35] collected subterranean termites, *Reticulitermes flavipes* and *Coptotermes formosanus*, using cardboard bait buried in the field infested with termites. For the same type of termites, El-Bassiouny et al. [36] used El-Sebay's [37] modified trap. Baimey et al. [31] broke at the top nests made by *T. occidentalis* and *M. bellicosus* in citrus orchards to collect directly workers and soldiers of the termites. Alternatively, these authors covered broken nests with dried straws. The straws were left well colonized by termites for 3–4 h and then termites were easily collected. For experiments designed to evaluate the nest reconstruction by termites following the break, it is advised to measure the height and surface denuded by the termites prior to breaking the nests.

Termites are usually collected in plastic containers, transferred to the laboratory where they are kept for given period of time before they are used for experiments. Authors of Refs. [31, 38] advised to put in the containers some moistened piece of paper as source of cellulose for the termites and also wet sand collected from termite nests. They also advised to keep the containers slightly open for aeration and in the dark at 25°C and 75–80% RH for 24 h before very active individuals are selected for experiments. El-Bassiouny et al. [36] rather kept termites at 25–28°C for 7 days in 9-cm diameter Petri dishes containing moistened corrugated cardboard before selecting active and vigorous individuals for use. Razia et al. [39] kept in the laboratory at 21–25°C workers of *R. flavipes* and *Odontotermis hornei* in plastic containers with 1–2 cm deep vermiculite sand and corrugated wood blocks added. Faye et al. [32] used sterilized soil (wetted soil heated to 80°C over a wood fire) on the surface of which vegetable debris was placed as culture media for *Odontotermes* spp.

2.5. Methods of control of termites

In response to the destructive activities of termites, man developed several preventative and remedial methods which are currently used against the pests [23]. Billions of dollars are spent annually throughout the world in this regard [26].

Chemical methods are practices frequently used against termites [40]. The methods rely on the use of synthetic chemicals such as dichloro diphenyl trichloroethane (DDT), benzene hexachloride (BHC), aldrin, dieldrin, soil barrier termiticides, dust and fumigant, treated zone termiticides [41]. These pesticides give quick control effects when they can reach termites but are costly, hazardous, and environmentally not safe. Therefore, despite this heavy reliance upon the application of chemical termiticides, future termite control technologies need to conform to higher environmental standards [7].

The most common nonchemical termite control method is the destruction of termite nests [42] because termites build epigeous mounds that affect cultivation and farm preparation [41]. This implies breaking and digging out the mound to reach and kill the reproductive queen and king of the nest [42]. But this method showed limitations as comeback is experienced after a period of time for some groups of termites that are capable of grooming new queen and king (*Cubitermes* and *Macrotermes*). Other nonchemical termite control methods include botanical termiticides [43], intercropping, crop rotation, planting of resistant crops [44], physical methods, i.e., debris removal, mechanical barriers, heat, high voltage electricity or electrocution, wood replacement, and biological control, i.e., use of predators [45], biological control agents such as fungi [46], bacteria, and nematodes [31, 35]. In a partial review, Myles [47] reported 2 viruses, 5 bacteria, 17 fungi, 5 nematodes, and 4 mites that have the potential to kill termites; the full list of these organisms being no doubt larger. But Weeks and Baker [48] reported that the behavior of termites affects the success of biological control. Lenz et al. [46] also reported that to be effective, biological control agents should be virulent, tolerate temperatures above 30°C, pose no health threats to man and higher animals, be easy mass produced and easy formulated, applied, and stored. Lacey et al. [49] observed that fast host killing ability, increased environmental persistence, long shelf life, good fitness into integrated systems, acceptance by growers, and general public are also parameters to consider. This book chapter will focus on the use of entomopathogenic nematodes as biological control agents against termites of economic importance in agriculture.

3. Entomopathogenic nematodes

3.1. Classification and distribution of entomopathogenic nematodes

Entomopathogenic nematodes (EPNs) are soil-inhabiting microorganisms. They have been isolated from all continents (except the Antarctic) and from a wide range of soil habitats: fields, forests, grasslands, desert, and ocean beaches [50]. They have been described from more than 40 nematode families. But only the Steinernematidae and Heterorhabditidae families have received the most attention because they possess several attributes of effective biological control agents [51, 52]. The family Steinernematidae contains two genera, i.e., *Steinernema* with more than 100 species and *Neosteinernema* with only one species, *Neosteinernema longicurvicauda* as parasite of termites [53]. The family Heterorhabditidae contains one genus, *Heterorhabditis*, with more than 20 species. The list of EPN species described in the world being too long, we give here only those reported from Africa. In Africa, to our knowledge, EPNs have been observed in Algeria, Benin, Cameroon, Egypt, Ethiopia, Kenya, Morocco, Nigeria, Rwanda, South Africa, and Tanzania (**Table 1**).

3.2. Advantages of the use of entomopathogenic nematode

Entomopathogenic nematodes have several distinct advantages over other forms of pest control in that they have a broad host range are easy to mass produce *in vivo* and *in vitro* [83] and to store. The use of EPNs for insect pest control is a rapid, sustainable, environmentally safe, and cost-effective method [84]. The nematodes can be applied with standard spray equipment in open environment [83, 85]. They are effective against a number of insect pests that occur in cryptic habitats including termites, having a high degree of safety among vertebrates and other non-target organisms [86]. Also, they have the potential to recycle in the environment, are amenable to genetic selection for desirable traits, and are exempt from registration in many countries [86, 87]. They are compatible with many chemical pesticides: herbicides, fungicides, acaricides, insecticides, nematicides [88–91], azadirachtin [92], *Bacillus thuringiensis* products, and pesticidal soap [93]. They are also compatible with many biological pesticides [86, 87] and with some parasitoids [49, 94]. Synergistic interaction between EPNs and other control agents has been observed for various insecticides [95, 96] and pathogens [97, 98].

3.3. Characteristics of entomopathogenic nematodes

Species of EPNs of the genera *Steinernema* and *Heterorhabditis* are successfully used to control insect pests. The IJs of the nematodes (the stage used as biopesticide) live symbiotically

Country	Species of entomopathogenic nematodes	References
Algeria	*S. feltiae*	[54, 55]
	H. bacteriophora	[55]
Benin	*Steinernema* sp, *H. sonorensis* and *H. indica*	[56, 57]
Cameroon	*H. amazoniensis, H. baujardi, S. cameroonense* and *S. nyetense*	[58]
Egypt	*H. indica, S. abbasi, S. carpocapsae, S. arenarium*	[59]
	H. baujardi	[60]
	H. bacteriophora, H. taysearae	[61]
Ethiopia	*S. ethiopiense*	[62]
	H. bacteriophora, and *S. yirgalemense*	[63]
Kenya	*H. bacteriophora, S. arenarium, S. glaseri*	[64]
	S. karii	[65]
	S. yirgalemense, S. weiserii, H. taysearae	[66]
	H. indica	[67]
Morocco	*S. feltiae*	[68]
Nigeria	*S. feltiae*	[69]
Rwanda	*S. carpocapsae* and *H. bacteriophora*	[70]
South Africa	*S. citrae; S. khoisanae; S. yirgalemense, H. zealandica* and *H.*	[71]
	bacteriophora	[72]
	S. khoisanae and H. bacteriophora	[73]
	H. safricana	[74]
	S. beitlechemi	[75]
	S. fabii	[76]
	S. innovationi	[77]
	S. jeffreyense	[78]
	S. sacchari	[79]
	S. tophus	[80]
	H. noenieputensis	[81]
	S. nguyeni	
Tanzania	*S. pwaniensis*	[82]

S. = *Steinernema*; *H.* = *Heterorhabditis*.

Table 1 Species of entomopathogenic nematodes isolated in Africa.

with bacteria of the genera *Xenorhabdus* and *Photorhabdus*, respectively [99]. They are nonfeeding and the only stage observed in the soil. They rely solely on energy reserves for survival and infectivity [100]. Their efficacy in the control of insect hosts is dependent on their attack strategy, survival, and persistence [101]. They use "sit and wait" (ambush foragers = most *Steinernema* nematodes), cruise (most *Heterorhabditis* nematodes), or intermediate foraging (some *Steinernema* nematodes) strategies to attack their insect hosts. Once inside the host haemocoel, the IJs of the nematodes release their symbiotic bacteria which proliferate and kill the host by septicemia within 48 h postinfection. Proliferated bacteria serve as source of food for the nematodes [102]. Also, these bacteria protect the host cadaver from colonization by other microorganisms including late arriving nematodes. Zhou et al. [103] reported that bacterial products from both *Xenorhabdus* and *Photorhabdus* make the infected insect repellent to ants. Fenton et al. [104] observed the protection of *Heterorhabditis bacteriophora*-infected cadavers from the avian predator, the European robin *Erithacus rubecula*. The authors reported that this protection was attributed to the red color reinforced by unpalatable taste of the cadavers and that the fact that the birds did not need to bite cadavers to reject them implies that some deterrent factor is emitted through the cadavers' cuticles. Thus, it is a nematode/bacterium complex that works together as a biological control unit to kill an insect host [85]. Insect susceptibility to EPN varies with insect species and is influenced by nematode species and strain [48]. Good knowledge of the IJs of EPNs and also of the relationships between IJs-insect-bacteria will allow increasing efficacy of treatment used to limit populations of pests [101]. Several researches are done in this regard using different protocols. The overall objective of these researches is to minimize pest populations to reduce losses they caused to crops. In countries where EPNs are observed and identified for the first time, researches usually start with the study of their biology under environmental extreme conditions in laboratory. This allows predicting which nematode isolate or species to use in target areas where environmental stress is expected.

3.4. Environmental stresses and their effect on the performance of entomopathogenic nematodes and their symbiotic bacteria

Authors of Refs. [48, 105] reported that the prevalence of infective juveniles (IJs) of EPNs in different habitats is affected by both intrinsic (behavioral, physiological, and genetic characteristics) and extrinsic (antibiotics, competition, natural enemies, temperature, soil moisture, pH, soil type, soil texture, relative humidity, UV radiation, and desiccation) factors. For experimental purposes, performance of EPNs is known by studying their ability to withstand conditions of drought, lack of oxygen, tolerance to heat [38, 106], capacity to search for targeted pests in the soil at specific concentration [107], to kill them, and to multiply inside them. The nematodes' tolerance to biotic factors is also studied under laboratory conditions. Most of the experiments designed in this regard are conducted using the larvae of the greater wax moth *Galleria mellonella* Linnaeus (Lepidoptera: Pyralidae), a model insect for EPN biology and pathogenicity studies [108]. Nematode isolates that perform best under laboratory conditions are then taken to semi-controlled and fields conditions [31, 36, 45] and tested against insect pests in biological control programs [31, 36, 106, 109, 110]. Grewal et al. [111] observed greatest performance of indigenous EPN isolates as compared to exotic ones for the control of insect pests for being used in their natural environment.

To evaluate the tolerance of IJs of indigenous EPNs to environmental stresses, the nematodes are subjected to temperatures varying between −5 and 40°C [38, 112–116], to hypoxia [38, 117], to dehydration/desiccation for up to 75% RH [118, 119], and to ultraviolet radiation stress (for example, at 340 nm, [120]). The persistence or longevity of indigenous EPN species in the soil [121], their genetic improvement, their infectivity [118, 119, 122], trehalose content/accumulation [123], motility, development, virulence, and reproduction inside insect hosts [124] under environmental stresses are some traits that are often evaluated. Antagonists [125], soil type [126], cultural conditions [127], and nematode species of strain [128] also affect nematode survival in soil. Studies on the symbiotic bacteria of EPNs include evaluation of growth and virulence of the bacteria under heat and cold temperatures [124]. All these different experiments are not only conducted mainly under laboratory [38, 106, 109, 118, 119] but also under greenhouse and field conditions [129, 130] either in open environments or in the dark [124].

The results from the different experiments are controversial and show variations for the potential of the nematode IJs to tolerate environmental stresses. This could be explained by differences among species and a great variability within species of EPNs, insect hosts, and also environmental stresses used in different experiments. Authors of Refs. [51, 131] reported moisture, temperature, foraging strategy, and pathogenicity for the targeted insect as the four most critical factors. Under adequate range of temperatures and moisture and with a susceptible host, EPNs with cruiser and intermediate foraging strategies are suitable for use in subterranean and certain aboveground habitats (foliar, epigeal, and cryptic habitats), while ambushers will be most effective in cryptic and soil surface habitats [132]. Authors of Refs. [122, 133] reported that temperatures of *ca.* 15–30°C provide highest and most stable survival (more than 95%) to nematodes' IJs than temperatures of *ca.* −5 to 10°C which reduce the nematodes' movement. Shapiro-Ilan et al. [134] reported significant contribution of the ability of EPNs to tolerate freezing conditions (−2°C for 6 or 24 h) to their biological control efficacy. But these authors did not observe any relationship between freezing and desiccation tolerance. This observation did not corroborate that of Solomon et al. [135] and Grewal et al. [136] who reported that tolerance to cold and desiccation is related in EPNs and that both stress factors cause an increase in trehalose levels, which is implicated as a physiological protectant. At high temperatures of *ca.* 35–40°C, nematode physiological activity is high, increasing the consumption of its stored energy and resulting in limited shelf life [112] and low searching [137] and pathogenicity [138] potential of the nematodes. Hang et al. [124] observed nematode IJs' development to adult at 13, 18, 24, 30, and 35°C and progeny production at 18, 24, and 30°C but not at 13 or 35°C. Zadji et al. [38] evaluated heat tolerance of 29 Benin isolates of *H. sonorensis* and one of *Heterorhabditis indica* under laboratory conditions using a method modified from Ref. [139]. Nematodes were subjected to 40°C for 2, 4, 6, and 8 h while being shaken at 70 rpm. The greatest survival of infective juveniles to heat (8 h), desiccation (8 h), and hypoxia (72 h) was observed with *H. sonorensis* isolates (72.8, 72.5, and 81.5%, respectively). Desiccation is important to conserve nematode IJ energy and improve their shelf life [140]. However, dehydration presents many challenges including difficulty in application because the carriers can block spray nozzles [141]. Genetic improvement of *H. bacteriophora* in beneficial traits as heat and desiccation tolerance by cross breeding and genetic selection is also reported. An overall increase in mean heat tolerance of 5.5°C by cross breeding five strains of the nematode species has been observed. But this enhanced heat tolerance and also tolerance to desiccation are often lost again during mass production. Fortunately, for Heterorhabditid nematodes, methods have now been developed to stabilize the traits by selection of tolerant inbred lines. This technique provides a pathway to genetic improvement of commercial strains which will maintain the improved characters also during *in vitro* mass production. For Steinernematid nematodes in contrast, the technique needs more investigation as these nematodes are amphimictic and production of inbred lines is much more laborious. Shapiro-Ilan et al. [139] reported that the effect of hypoxia on nematode IJs' survival varied significantly with duration of exposure of the nematodes to stressed conditions and with nematode isolates from 33.2 to 81.5% and from 85.9 to 96.9% after 24 and 72 h of exposure, respectively. Entomopathogenic nematodes are sensitive to UV light. This is why they are usually applied to protected environments, particularly soil [86, 142]. But extended persistence of nematode IJs in the soil results in greater cumulative insect host mortality and reduced need for multiple nematode applications.

3.5. Mass production of entomopathogenic nematodes for laboratory and field application

Before EPN isolates with desirable characteristics such as tolerance to environmental stresses and virulence to insect hosts are used for experiments or for commercialization [143], they are cultured *in vivo* or *in vitro* at a small scale [144] or at a large scale [145].

3.5.1. In vivo production

For laboratory use and small-scale field experiments, *in vivo* production of EPNs appears to be appropriate method. Though various caterpillars and large beetle larvae are very susceptible insects to EPNs, for most laboratories and some field experiments, EPNs are mostly reared in last instar larvae of the greater wax moth, *G. mellonella* as described by Kaya et al. [144]. The larvae of *G. mellonella* can be produced using an artificial medium containing 22% ground wheat, 22% ground maize, 11% honey, 11% glycerol, 11% milk powder, 5.5% yeast extract, and 17.5% bee wax in a glass jar at 25°C in the laboratory [146]. The larvae of this insect are preferred because they are very susceptible to the nematodes and very easy to mass rear, they are commonly sold as fish bait. Nematode-infected larvae are incubated for around 72 h at 25-27°C before being transferred onto White trap. Hundreds of thousands of IJs of the nematodes emerge from infected *G. mellonella* larvae as progeny in few days [31, 109]. Emerged nematodes are collected [36, 39, 106] and used immediately [31] for experiments. They may be stored in tissue culture flask at 13°C [36, 115, 147] or at 19°C [39] and are used within 5 days [36, 39] or 2–6 weeks [109, 145] after collection. Though *in vivo* production of EPN is simple, reliable and results in high quality nematodes, the method is labor intensive and costly.

3.5.2. In vitro production

In vitro method of nematode production is used when large-scale production is needed at reasonable quality and cost. Two methods are used for *in vitro* production of EPN, i.e., solid media and liquid fermentation [148, 149]. The first method uses crumbed polyether polyurethane foam coated with a nutritive medium and inoculated first with symbiotic bacteria and then with nematodes. This method requires limited experience, its capital costs are low and logistics of production is flexible. The liquid fermentation method has the lowest mass production cost and is used by large companies with multiple products. The method relies on suitable medium composed of yeast extract as nitrogen source, a carbohydrate source as soy flour, glucose, or glycerol, lipids of plant or animal origin and salts and requires adequate oxygen [150, 151]. The following EPN species have been successfully produced using liquid fermentation method with yield capacity as high as 250,000 infective juveniles/ml: *Steinernema*

http://dx.doi.org/10.5772/intechopen.69861

carpocapsae, Steinernema riobrave, Steinernema kushidai, Steinernema feltiae, Steinernema glaseri, Steinernema scapterisci, H. bacteriophora, and *Heterorhabditis megidis* in 7500–80,000 liter bioreactors. Ehlers [152] reported that industrial-scale *in vivo* EPN production is applicable in developing countries and the large-scale *in vitro* production best suited for countries with low labor costs or for serving high value markets.

3.6. Storage and formulation of entomopathogenic nematodes

When nematodes are not to be used immediately, they are kept in appropriate conditions for a while to avoid their deterioration. Several methods are used to store EPNs for extended periods or to formulate them immediately following their mass production. But before they are stored or formulated for successful control of insect pests, the quality (i.e., viability based on their movement, energy reserves, and infectivity) of IJs of the nematodes is checked. Authors of Refs. [100, 153] reported the one-on-one (one nematode to one *G. mellonella* larvae) sand-well assay. The energy reserves (dry weight and total lipid content) are predictors of nematode longevity. Because each nematode species has its specific requirements for temperature, moisture and oxygen [112, 140, 154, 155], it becomes difficult to obtain a formulation or storage condition suitable for all EPN species. Nematodes are stored on moist sponge, in formulations that contain alginate, vermiculite, clays, activated charcoals, polyacrylamide, and water dispersible granules or are partially desiccated in water dispersible granules [88, 149]. To be successful, any formulation method should consider reducing nematode metabolism by immobilization or partial desiccation. *Steinernema* species can be stored in aqueous suspension for 6–12 months at 4–15°C, while *Heterorhabditis* species can be stored only for 3–6 months at the same temperature. Partially-desiccated infective juveniles in water dispersible granules have a shelf life of 5–6 months for *S. carpocapsae* at 25°C and 2 months for *S. feltiae,* and 1 month for *S. riobrave* [156] at the same temperature.

3.7. Quality control of entomopathogenic nematodes

Before EPNs are used in the laboratory or in the field after being stored or formulated, they are acclimated at room temperature of *ca.* 25°C for 2 h. Their quality is then checked again, and their concentrations to be used in experiments are adjusted by volumetric dilutions in distilled water using the formula as given in Ref. [157].

4. Control of termites using entomopathogenic nematodes and their symbiotic bacteria

Authors of Refs. [158, 159] first reported the presence of parasitic head inhabiting nematodes in the termites *Reticulitermes lucifugus* and *C. formosanus*. But only 40 years later, Tamashiro [160] first proposed the use of nematodes against termites. Control of the pest based on the use of EPNs became a promising technology for future termite control option. Since then, a plethora of laboratory and in some extent field research efforts resulting in subsequent publications on biological control of termites have been observed [83, 161–164].

4.1. Control under laboratory conditions

Several experiments showed the effectiveness of EPNs to control termites under laboratory conditions. In the laboratory, bioassays with termites and EPNs are usually carried out in containers such as Petri dishes lined with wet filter paper or sterile sand [39, 109], PCV tubes, or Eppendorf tubes [109]. In all cases, piece of filter paper [165], straw [106], and also corrugated wood blocks [39] are usually used in the containers to serve as food for termites [48]. Nematodes strains used for inoculations are usually selected from a number of strains based on their greater virulence to *G. mellonella* larvae [39]. Selected strains are then mass reared [144] to have sufficient inoculums. Each container receives given population densities of nematodes, most of the time in the form of water suspension with appropriate water volumes. In the case of low population densities, nematodes are transferred into the containers using micropipettes [165].

According to the objectives of the experiment, termite castle (reproductive adults, soldiers, or workers) or developmental stage (larvae, nymphs, and adults) is selected and transferred into containers following nematode introduction [36]. Host-finding ability and nematode virulence (ability of the nematodes to kill their host and to produce offspring inside them) are recorded. Nematode mortality is recorded daily or at given intervals of time following inoculation to evaluate lethal dose (LD_{10}, LD_{50}, or LD_{90}) and lethal time (LT_{10}, LT_{50}, or LT_{90}). Insects that are killed are dissected 48 h postinoculation in Ringer solution under stereo-microscope to confirm parasitism and to record population density of infecting nematodes inside each termite and developmental stage of the nematodes. Also, part of termites killed by the nematodes is transferred to White traps (i.e., emerging from hosts and accumulating in water) for days to evaluate nematode progeny production [39, 109]. Because termites are very fragile, some usually die naturally during the course of the experiments. In this case, insect mortality data are corrected using the following formula of Ref. [166]: $Mc = [(Mo - Mc')/(100-Mc')] \times 100$, where Mc = corrected mortality, Mo = Mortality caused by the nematodes, Mc′ = Mortality observed in control treatments.

Wang et al. [35] showed that *S. carpocapsae* and *H. bacteriophora* were effective against workers of the subterranean termite *R. flavipes under laboratory conditions*. The same authors also reported that *H. indica* was more efficient than both *S. carpocapsae* and *H. bacteriophora* against *R. flavipes*. Razia et al. [39] studied in sand assay method the virulence of *S. siamkayai, S. pakistanense,* and *H. indica* applied at 100, 250, 300, 500, 700, and 900 IJs/ml suspension on workers of subterranean termites, *R. flavipes* and *O. hornei* (25 termites/Petri dish). The authors observed positive relationship between concentration and exposure time and mortality and variation between nematode and termite species for LD_{10}, LT_{50}, and LT_{90}. El-Sebay et al. [36] conducted similar experiment using Egyptian isolates of *Heterorhabditis baujardi* and *H. indica* to control *Psammotermes hypostoma* and *Anacanthotermes ochraceus* under laboratory conditions. The authors observed LC_{50} and LC_{90} values of, respectively, 15.03 and 361.53 for *P. hypostoma* and *H. baujardi* and 20.26 and 398.59 for *H. baujardi* and *A. ochraceus* at day 3 after inoculation. For the experiment, highest rate of insect mortality was observed at day 3 after inoculation. Zadji et al. [38] tested in 2-ml Eppendorf tubes (each with 50 nematodes and 1 insect) the pathogenicity of 29 Benin isolates of H. *sonorensis* and one H. *indica* against workers of M. *bellicosus*. The results of the experiment showed that 73% of the nematode isolates killed more than 80% of the insects. In another study, Zadji et al. [106] evaluated the differential susceptibility of workers and soldiers of two termite species, *M. bellicosus* and *T. occidentalis*, to four Benin isolates of EPNs: one *H. indica*, two *H. sonorensis*, and one *Steinernema* sp. (5, 10, 25, 50, or 100 nematodes/well of tissue culture plates with one insect). A significant difference in termite mortality was recorded between termite castes but not between EPN isolates and termite species. Soldiers of both *M. bellicosus* and *T. occidentalis* were similarly susceptible but more susceptible than workers. The LD_{50} varied with termite species and nematode isolates from 12 IJs (*T. occidentalis* with *Steinernema* sp.) to 23 IJs (*M. bellicosus* with *Steinernema* sp.).

The reproduction potential of EPNs inside termites varies not only with nematode species but also with termite species and caste. Zadji et al. [109] observed up to 20,213 *H. sonorensis* IJs per worker of *M. bellicosus* 10 days postinoculation with an average of six nematodes penetrating each insect. Wang et al. [35] similarly, but in much lower population densities, observed an average number of IJs of 289 ± 50 and 642 ± 93 per worker, respectively, produced from *R. flavipes* and *C. formosanus* (based on 11 and 8 workers, respectively). The nematodes were seen through the cuticle of dead termites 4–5 days postinoculation, and they began to emerge at day 5 after infestation. The authors concluded that EPNs have the potential to continue their infestation to termites after an initial treatment. But in the same experiments, they observed consumption of some nematode-killed termites by healthy termites or by a saprophagous mite, *Australhypopus* sp. This mite is very common on the body of *R. flavipes*, especially on the head. Once the termite dies, the mite reproduces quickly in large numbers and feeds on the dead termite. The consumption of dead termites by healthy ones and also by *Australhypopus* sp. is a cause for the failure of nematode recycling in termites.

Some others experiments are designed to evaluate the potential of the nematodes' symbiotic bacteria to kill termites or to evaluate the efficacy of combined effect of nematodes with other insect control methods on termites. *H. bacteriophora* and their associated bacteria were found to be effective against workers and nymphs of six different species of termites: *C. formosanus, Gnathamitermes perplexus, Heterotermes aureus, P. hybostoma, R. flavipes,* and *R. virginicus*. Meanwhile, *H. indica* and *Photorhabdus luminescens* complex were found to be effective against three species of termites: *C. formosanus, C. vastator,* and *R. flavipes*. *S. carpocapsae* together with their symbiotic bacteria, *X. nematophila,* are capable of suppressing population of eight different termite species including *C. formosanus, C. vastator, G. perplexus, H. aureus, P. hybostoma, R. flavipes, R. virginicus,* and *Zootermopsis angusticollis*.

Two-container choice device is used to evaluate the repellency of nematodes to termites [35] as described by Mauldin and Beal [167]. Wang et al. [35] used this method to study the repellency of four EPNs: *S. carpocapsae, Steinernema riobrave, H. bacteriophora,* and *H. indica* to two subterranean termites: *R. flavipes* and *C. formosanus*. *H. indica* repelled termites at high concentrations (90 nematodes/cm^3 and above) in sand and vermiculite medium. The length of repellency varied (from 3 to 17 days postinoculation) with the nematode concentration and the size of the device used for the experiment. Similar experiment was conducted by Zadji et al. [106] with Benin nematode isolates: one *H. indica,* two *H. sonorensis,* and one *Steinernema* sp. (962.5 nematode IJs/cm^3 of 40 cm^3 sterilized sand) and termite species, *M. bellicosus* and *T.*

occidentalis. The experiment did not show evidence that *M. bellicosus* and *T. occidentalis* would be able to detect the presence of IJs of any EPN isolates. However, it was observed that nematode dispersal occurred by infected termites or phoresis.

The results of these experiments showed that, usually, under laboratory conditions, pathogenicity of nematodes to termites is certain as the host contact is certain, environmental conditions are optimal and no ecological or behavioral barriers to infection exist [168]. But under field conditions, successful termite control using nematodes is less certain.

4.2. Control under field conditions

In the world in general and in Africa in particular, field studies on the use of EPNs to control termites are limited [31, 169]. The few studies compared the effects of various formulations and methods of applications of the nematodes on the mortality of different casts and life stages of termites evaluated the performance of different nematode isolates on the progress of termite nests' reconstruction, the persistence of the nematodes in the nests, the percentage of nests for which the underground termite populations died, and the progeny production of the nematodes inside their host [31]. The ability of termites to detect the nematodes and to avoid them [48], and the overall behavior of termites following colonization of the nests by nematodes were also studied. The advantage of the use of EPNs over other methods, especially over chemical methods, for the control of termites under field conditions, is the capacity of nematodes to reach cryptic habitat of termites, difficultly reachable by chemical pesticides; termites live in an environment conducive to nematodes. A wide range of EPNs were identified in this regard as effective against various termite species [26, 31] under field conditions. But the nematode formulation used affects the success of the pest control.

Nematode water suspension (i.e., nematodes in water) or nematode-infected *G. mellonella* larvae are two nematode formulations mostly used in the fields to control termites [31, 46, 83]. In the case of nematode suspension, the nematode inoculum is applied using common nozzle type sprayers (hand and ground sprayers) with openings as small as 100 μm in diameter and with pressure of up to 1068 kPa on nematodes [170] in the field or using simple water cans on small areas against termites [171] successfully controlled *Neotermes* sp. associated with coconut palms and citrus trees. Meanwhile, Lenz et al. [172] injected *Heterorhabditis indicus* into cavity of mahogany tree against *Neotermes* sp. Also, Gouge [83] and Lenz [46] injected nematodes in tree trunks to control *Mastotermes darwiniensis* using *Heterorhabditis* sp. But the authors reported that the success of termite control is affected by the plant structure. For example, it is difficult to apply nematodes to the entire termite colony of branched trees, where termites find refuge in untreated branches of the plant.

For successful termite control, especially with nematode-infected *G. mellonella* larvae, the aboveground termite nests are first demolished before nematode suspension or infected *G. mellonella* larvae are applied. Baimey et al. [31] applied 52-week-old EPN-infected *G. mellonella* larvae per nest, each larva containing *ca.* 200,000 of IJs of Benin isolates of *H. sonorensis* and *H. indica*. At day 70 after inoculation, the underground populations of 71 and 60% treated nests were controlled by *H. sonorensis* and *H. indica*-infected *G. mellonella* larvae, respectively. When applied in infected *G. mellonella* larvae, nematodes will be protected for a while against environmental stresses before emerging from the larvae and will certainly provide superior termite control as compared to nematodes applied in water suspension which will be rapidly affected by environmental stresses soon after their application.

Termite workers are able to reconstruct their nest after this is broken. Baimey et al. [31] reported that nest reconstruction as measured by the nest reconstruction rate (see formula below) differed significantly among nematode isolates and time of exposure of inocula to termites with significant correlation between the two parameters. The nest reconstruction rate (NRR) is estimated as followed: NRR = $(V_n/V_0) \times 100$, where V_n is the aboveground reconstructed nest volume *n* days after application of EPN-infected *G. mellonella* larvae and V_0 the volume of the aboveground nest before its demolition. The nest volume is calculated using the formula to calculate the volume of a cone, $V = 1/3\pi \times R^2 \times h$, where *R* (m) is the nest radius and *h* (m) the nest height.

Even though termite nest can be reconstructed after being broken or after nematode application, nematode persistence in the nest area is necessary to avoid frequent breaks and also frequent applications of the nematodes for successful control of termites. Nematode persistence in the nest can be assessed by randomly taking soil samples from treated nest at intervals of days and by baiting the samples with last instars *G. mellonella* larvae. Baimey et al. [31] took nest samples 10, 20, and 70 days postinoculation. The samples were baited with *G. mellonella* larvae for a week at 25 ± 1°C and dead larvae recorded daily from the 5th day to the 7th day. Cadavers of *G. mellonella* larvae were dissected to confirm EPN infection. Susurluk et al. [173] stated that the number of infected larvae found by sampling is related to the number of nematodes that were present in the soil.

Authors of Refs. [48, 174] reported an ability of some termite species (example of *Reticulitermes tibialis*) to detect EPN and avoid them or to detect other termites that have died from nematode infection. Nematode-killed individuals are walled off to avoid or reduce contamination to other individuals in the nest [175, 176]. Authors of Refs. [169, 177] stated that though nematodes appear to have a limited impact on subterranean and dampwood termites due to termite behavioral defense mechanisms, they successfully control drywood termites where colonies are contained within a single piece of wood or a single tree. Similarly, Fujii [178] reported that this walling-off behavior of certain termite species does not prevent the dispersal of nematodes inside the occlusion as, at least, nematodes that were produced from partially or loosely buried termites are often observed outside the occlusion. Wang et al. [35] reported a repellence of EPNs to termites and concluded that the repellence might be the main reason for the ineffectiveness of nematodes to termites in certain field experiments. Therefore, it is important to consider the species of termites before selecting the EPN isolates.

5. Limitations in the use of entomopathogenic nematodes as biological control agents of termites

The various information given in this chapter indicated that EPNs provides some successful control of termite. But the method presents some limitations that should be taken into account.

An example of limitation is the high nematode population densities needed for successful control of termites: approximately 23,000 infective juveniles of *H. bacteriophora, S. carpocapsae,* and *S. feltiae* nematodes are required to treat one square foot of termite infested area. Authors of Refs. [179, 180] stated that for successful control of drywood termites, all portions of the gallery system need to be located and treated. Nematodes were effective on the dampwood termite in the genus *Neotermes* infesting unbranched trunks of coconut palms, but their effectiveness was inferior in branched trees of citrus, cocoa, or mahogany [172]. The high numbers of termites in a nest, the wide foraging range of termites, the limited mobility of nematodes, the low reproduction rate of some nematode isolates in dead termites, and the repellence of some nematodes to termites are other examples of limitations for successful control of termites by nematodes, especially in field conditions. In this regard, Wang et al. [35] advised inundative release of EPNs rather than classical biological control for the control of subterranean termites. To increase termite susceptibility to EPNs, some researchers refer to sublethal doses of chemical termiticides, other biological control agents as fungi [181, 182] and bacteria [98] and imidacloprid [95, 183, 184] in an integrated pest management programs. However, this method encounters the problem of delivery of those insecticides to termite individuals at a distance from the application site [185]. Moreover, the method needs to provide cost effective protection against termite damage [35]. Temperatures of above 30°C in the center of the nests of *Coptotermes* species, where reproductives and brood are housed, are lethal for the nematodes. This means that different isolates or species of EPNs that are tolerant to higher temperatures are required for subterranean termite species. The diffuse nest system, the presence of multiple sets of reproductives, large territory size, and simultaneous use of many feeding sites also make the successful control of some termite species using EPNs difficult. Weeks and Baker [48] reported that the nematodes must be placed in environments congenial to their survival or they prove useless for control. More studies are then needed on these limitations for easier and better control of termites using EPNs.

Acknowledgements

The Flemish Inter-University Council-University Development Co-operation (VLIR-UOS), Belgium funded the first soil samplings for EPNs in Benin and also the first research activities on the control of citrus termites using Beninese isolates of nematodes through the *"Ecological Sustainable Citrus Production in Benin"* Project. VLIR-UOS is gratefully acknowledged by the authors of this paper.

Author details

Hugues Baïmey[1]*, Lionel Zadji[1], Léonard Afouda[1], André Fanou[1], Régina Kotchofa[1] and Wilfrieda Decraemer[2]

*Address all correspondence to: baimeyhugues@gmail.com

1 University of Parakou, Benin

2 Ghent University, Belgium

References

[1] Grimaldi D, Engel MS. Evolution of the Insects. Cambridge University Press; Cambridge, UK. 2005. p. 145. ISBN-13 978-0-521-82149-0 hardback, ISBN-10 0-521-82149-5 hardback

[2] AbeT, BignellDE, HigashiM. Termites: Evolution, Socially, Symbioses, Ecology. Dordrecht/ Norwell: Kluwer Academic Publishers; 2000. p. 56. DOI: 10.1007/978-94-017-3223-9

[3] Ohiagu CE. Nest and soil population of *Trinervitermes* spp. with particular reference to *Trinervitermes germinatus* (Wasmann), Isoptera in Southern Guinea Savanna near Mokwa, Nigeria. Oecologia. 1979;**40**(2):167-178. DOI: 100.1007/BF00347934

[4] Harris WV. Termites of the Palearctic Region. In: Krishna K, Weesner FM, editors. Biology of Termites Ville et Pays?; Kluwer Academic Publishers, Dordrecht, The Netherlands. 1970. pp. 2:295-2:313. ISBN-10: 012426302X, ISBN-13: 978-0124263024

[5] Engel MS, Krishna K. Family-group names for Termites (Isoptera). American Museum Novitates. 2004;**3432**:1-9. DOI: 10.1206/0003-0082(2004)432<0001:FNFTI>2.0.CO;2

[6] Vargo EL, Husseneder C. Biology of subterranean termite: Insights from molecular studies of *Reticulitermes* and *Coptotermes*. Annual Review of Entomology. 2009;**54**:379-403. DOI: 10.1146/annurev.ento.54.110807.090443

[7] Su N-Y. Novel technologies for subterranean termite control. Sociobiology. 2002;**40** (1):95-101

[8] Adams BJ, Fodor A, Koppenhöfer HS, Stackenbrandt E, Stock SP, Klein MG. Biodiversity and systematic of nematode–bacterium entomopathogens. Biological Control. 2006;**37**: 32-49. DOI: 10.1016/j.biocontrol.2005.11.008

[9] Chouvenc T, Su N-Y, Grace JK. Fifty years of attempted biological control of termites – Analysis of a failure. Biological Control. 2011;**59**:69-82. DOI: 10.1016/j.biocontrol.2011.06.015

[10] Baker PB, Marchosky RJ. Arizona Termites of Economic Importance. Tucson, AZ: University of Arizona Press; 2005. p. 20

[11] Grohmann C, Oldeland J, Stoyan D, Linsenmair KE. Multi-scale pattern analysis of a mound building Termite Species. Insectes Sociaux. 2010;**57**(4):367-494. ISBN: 978-84-608-8178-0

[12] Kambhampati S, Eggleton P. Taxonomy and phylogeny of termites. In: Abe Y, Bignell DE, Higsahi M, editors. Termites: Evolution, Sociality, Symbioses, Ecology. The Netherlands: Kluwer Academic Publishers, Dordrecht; 2000. pp. 1-23. DOI: 10.1007/978-94-017-3223-9_1

[13] Engel MS. Family-group names for termites (Isoptera), redux. In: Engel MS, editor. Contributions Celebrating Kumar Krishna. ZooKeys; Pensoft Publishers. Sofia, Bulgaria; 2011. pp. 171-184. DOI: 10.3897/zookeys.148.1682

[14] Ahmed BM, Nkunika POY, Sileshi GW, French JRJ, Nyeko P, Jain S. Potential impact of climate change on termite distribution in Africa. British Journal of Environment and Climate Change. 2011;**1**(4):172-189. DOI: 10.9734/BJECC/2011/561

[15] Kanwal HK, Acharya K, Ramesh G, Reddy MS. Molecular characterization of *Morchella* species from the Western Himalayan region of India. Current Microbiology. 2011;**62**(4):1245-1252. DOI: 10.1007/s00284-010-9849-1

[16] Eggleton P. Global patterns of termite diversity. In: Abe T, Bignell DE, Higashi M, editors. Termites: Evolution, Sociality, Symbioses, Ecology. Dordrecht: Kluwer; 2000. pp. 25-51. DOI: 10.1007/978-94-017-3223-9

[17] Eggleton P. Termite species description rates and the state of termite taxonomy. Insects Sociaux. 1999;**46**:1-5. DOI: 10.1007/s000400050105

[18] Mahaney WC, Zippin J, Milner MW, Sanmugadas K, Hancock RGV, Aufreiter S, Kalm V. Chemistry, mineralogy and microbiology of termite mound soil eaten by the chimpanzees of the Mahale Mountains, Western Tanzania. Journal of Tropical Ecology. 1999;**15**(05):565-588

[19] Kemabonta KA, Balogun SA. Species richness, diversity and relative abundance of termites (Insecta-Isoptera) in the University of Lagos, Lagos Nigeria. FUTA Journal of Resesrch in Sciences. 2014;**2**:188-197. ISSN: 2315-8239

[20] Kleis R. Van huis figures out cultural significance of termites. 2017. Science. Available from: https://resource.wur.nl/en/science/show/Van-Huis-figures-out-cultural-significance-of-termites.htm

[21] Reis de Figueirêdo REC, Vasconcellos A, Policarpo IS, Alves RRN. Edible and medicinal termites: A global overview. Journal of Ethnobiology and Ethnomedicine. 2015;**11**:29. DOI: 10.1186/s13002-015-0016-4

[22] Okonya JS, Kroschler J. Indigenous knowledge of seasonal weather forecasting. A case study of six regions of Uganda. Agricultural Sciences. 2013;**4**(12):641-648. DOI: 10.4236/as.2013.412086

[23] Su N-Y, Scheffrahn RH. Termites as pests of buildings. In: Abe T, Bignell DE, Higashi M, editors. Termites: Evolution, Sociality, Symbiosis, Ecology. Dordrecht/Norwell: Kluwer Academic; 2000. pp. 437-453. DOI: 10.1007/978-94-017-3223-9

[24] Lee KE, Wood TG. Termites and Soils. London, UK: Academic Press; 1971. pp. 65-71. ISBN: 0124408508

[25] Cowie RH, Logan JWM, Wood TG. Termite (Isoptera) damage and control in tropical forestry with special reference to Africa and Indo-Malaysia: A review. Bulletin of Entomological Research. 1989;**79**(2):173-184. DOI: https://doi.org/10.1017/S0007485300018150

[26] Khan MA, Ahmad W, Paul B, Paul S, Khan Z, Aggarwal C. Entomopathogenic nematodes for the management of subterranean termites. In: Hakeem KR, Akhtar MS, Abdullah SNA, editors. Plant, Soil and Microbes. Vol. 1. Switzerland: Implications in Crop Science. Springer International Publishing; 2016. pp. 317-352. DOI: 10.1007/978-3-319-27455-3_16

[27] Traniello JFA, Leuthold RH. Behavior and ecology of foraging in termites. In: Abe T, Bignell DE, Higashi M, editors. Termites: Evolution, Sociality, Symbioses, Ecology. Dordrecht: Kluwer; 2000. pp. 141-168. DOI: 10.1007/978-94-017-3223-9_7

[28] Dangerfield JM, McCarthy TS, Ellery WN. The mound-building termite *Macrotermes michaelseni* as an ecosystem engineer. Journal of Tropical Ecology. 1998;**14**(4):507-520. pISSN: 0266-4674, e-ISSN: 1469-7831

[29] Available from: http://www.articles.nydailynews.com/2011-04-25/news/29492144_1_rupee_state_bank_termites. [Acessed: 12 May 2017]

[30] Ecologically Sustainable Citrus Production in Benin (ESCiP – Benin). Annual Activity Report. Benin: University of Parakou; 2015. p. 32

[31] Baimey H, Zadji L, Afouda L, Moens M, Decraemer W. Influence of pesticides, soil temperature and moisture on entomopathogenic nematodes from southern Benin and control of underground termite nest populations. Nematology. 2015;**17**:1057-1069. DOI: 10.1163/15685411-00002923

[32] Faye A, Kane PD, Mbaye DF, Sall Sy D, Sane D. Study of the cassava varietal sensitivity to termites ravaging cuttings planted in farms in the department of Tivaouane (Senegal). International Journal of Science and Advanced Technology. 2014;**46**(6):6-16. ISSN: 2221-8386

[33] Riekert HF, Van den Berg J. Evaluation of chemical control measures for termites in maize. South African Journal of Plant Soil. 2003;**20**:1-5. DOI:10.1080/02571862.2003.10634896

[34] Kumar D, Pardeshi M. Biodiversity of termites in agro-ecosystem and relation between their niche breadth and pest status. Journal of Entomology. 2011;**8**:250-258. DOI: 10.3923/je.2011.250.258

[35] Wang C, Powell JE, Nguyen K. Laboratory evaluations of four entomopathogenic nematodes for control of subterranean termites (Isoptera: Rhinotermitidae). Environmental Entomology. 2002;**31**(2):381-387. DOI: http://dx.doi.org/10.1603/0046-225X-31.2.381

[36] El-Bassiouny RR, Randa M. Susceptibility of Egyptian subterranean termite to some entomopathogenic nematodes. Egyptian Journal of Agricultural Research. 2011;**89**(1):121-135. ISSN: 1110-6336

[37] El-Sebay Y. A modified trap for El-Sebay subterranean termites. Fourth Arabian Congress of Plant Protection, Cairo, 1-5 December 1991. 111, 1991

[38] Zadji L, Baimey H, Afouda L, Moens M, Decraemer W. Characterization of biocontrol traits of heterorhabditid entomopathogenic nematode isolates from South Benin targeting the termite pest *Macrotermes bellicosus*. BioControl. 2014;**59**(3):333-344. DOI: 10.1007/s10526-014-9568-9

[39] Razia M, Sivaramakrishnan S. Evaluation of *Entomopathogenic* nematodes against Termites. Journal of Entomology and Zoology Studies. 2016;**4**(4):324-327. eISSN: 2320-7078; pISSN: 2349-6800

[40] HDRA – The Organic Organisation. Termite Control Without Chemicals. UK: HDRA Publishing; 2001. p. 16

[41] Ibrahim BU, Adebote DA. Appraisal of the economic activities of termites: A review. Bayero Journal of Pure and Applied Sciences. 2012;**5**(1):84-89. DOI: http://dx.doi.org/10.4314/bajopas.v5i1.16

[42] Mugerwa S, Mpairwe D, Zziwa E, Sawaans K, Peden D. Integrated Termite Management for Improved Rainwater Management. A Synthesis of Selected African Experiences. NBDC Technical Report-9. 2014

[43] Verma M, Sharma S, Prasad R. Biological alternative for termite control: A review. International Biodeterioration and Biodegradation. 2009;**63**:959-972. DOI: 10.1016/j.ibiod.2009.05.009

[44] UNEP (United Nations Environment Program). Finding Alternative Methods to Persistent Organic Pollutants (Pops) for the Termite Management. UNEP/FAO/Globa l IPM Facility Expert Group on Termite Biology and Management. Nairobi, Kenya. 2000. p. 50. Available from: https://nature.berkeley.edu/upmc/documents/UN_termite.pdf

[45] Culliney TW, Grace JK. Prospects for the biological control of subterranean termites (Isoptera: Rhinotermitidae), with special reference to *Coptotermes formosanus*. Bulletin of Entomological Research. 2000;**29**(1):9-21 DOI: 10.1017/S0007485300000031

[46] Lenz M. Biological control in termite management: The potential of nematodes and fungal pathogens. In: Lee CY, Robinson WH, editors. Proceedings of the Fifth International Conference on Urban Pests. Singapore, 10-13 July 2005. Perniagaan Ph'ng @ P&Y Design Network, Penang, Malaysia; 2005. pp. 47-52

[47] Myles TG. Isolation of *Metarhizium anisopliae* (Deuteromycotina: Hyphomycetes) from *Reticulitermes flavipes* (Isoptera: Rhinotermitdae) with convenient methods for its culture and collection of conidia. Sociobiology. 2002;**40**(2):257-264. ISSN: 0361-6525

[48] Weeks B, Baker P. Subterranean Termite (Isoptera: Rhinotermitidae) Mortality Due to Entomopathogenic Nematodes (Nematoda: Steinernematidae, Heterorhabditidae). University of Arizona College of Agriculture. Turfgrass and Ornamental Research Report, Index available from: http://cals.arizona.edu/pubs/crops/az1359/. 2004. pp. 1-5

[49] Lacey LA, Frutos R, Kaya HK, Vail P. Insect pathogens as biological control agents: Do they have a future? Biological Control. 2001;**21**:230-248. DOI: 10.1006/bcon.2001.0938

[50] Poinar GO. Taxonomy and biology of Steinernematidae and Heterorhabditidae. In: Gaugler R, Kaya H, editors. Entomopathogenic nematodes in biological control. Boca Raton: CRC Press, Florida; 1990. 23-61

[51] Grewal PS, Ehlers R-U, Shapiro-Ilan DI. Nematodes as Biological Control Agents. Wallingford, UK: CABI Publishing; 2005. p. 528. DOI: 10.1079/9780851990170.0000

[52] Koppenhöfer AM. Nematodes. In: Lacey LA, Kaya HK, editors. Field Manual of Techniques in Invertebrate Pathology: Application and Evaluation of Pathogens for Control of Insects and Other Invertebrate Pests, 2nd ed. Dordrecht: Springer; 2007. pp. 249-264. DOI: 10.1007/978-1-4020-5933-9

[53] Nguyen KB, Smart GC. Scanning electron microscope studies of spicules and gubernacula of *Steinernema* spp. (Nemata: Steinernematidae). Nematologica. 1997;**43**:465-480. DOI: 10.1163/005125997X00066

[54] Tarasco E, Triggiani O, Sai K, Zanoum M. Survey on entomopathogenic nematodes in Algerian soils and their activity at different temperatures. Frustula Entomologica. 2009;**32**(45):31-42

[55] Zamoum M, Berchiche S, Sai K, Triggiani O, Tarasco E. Preliminary survey of the occurrence of Entomopathogenic Nematodes and fungi in the forest soils of Algeria. Silva Lusitana. 2011;**19**:141-145

[56] Zadji L, Baimey H, Afouda L, Houssou GF, Waeyenberge L, de Sutter N, Moens M, Decraemer W. First record on the distribution of entomopathogenic nematodes (Rhabditida: Steinernematidae and Heterorhabditidae) in Southern Benin. Russian Journal of Nematology. 2013; **21**(2):117-130. ISSN : 0869-6918

[57] Houssou GF, Baimey H, Zadji L, de Sutter N, Waeyenberge L, Afouda L, Viane N, Moens M, Decraemer W. Taxonomic study of entomopathogenic nematodes (Nematoda: Steinernematidae, Heterorhabditidae) from Benin. *Agronomie Africaine*. 2014;**26**(3):231-245. ISSN: 1015-2288

[58] Kanga FN, Waeyenberge L, Hauser S, Moens M. Distribution of entomopathogenic nematodes in Southern Cameroon. Journal of Invertebrate Pathology. 2012;**109**:41-51. DOI: 10.1016/j.jip.2011.09.008

[59] Abd-Elbary NA, Shamseldean MSM, Stock SP, Abu-Shady NM. Diversity of entomopathogenic nematode species (Heterorhabditidae and Steinernematidae) in Egypt. Egyptian Journal of Agronematology. 2012;**11**(2):333-353. ISSN: 1110-6158

[60] Abd El-Rahman RM. Isolation and identification of *Heterorhabditis baujardi* as a first record from Egypt and studying some of its biological traits. Egyptian Journal of Applied Science. 2006;**8**(2A):298-307

[61] Abd-Elgawad MMM, Nguyen KB. Isolation, identification and environmental tolerance of new heterorhabditid populations from Egypt. International Journal of Nematology. 2007;**17**(2):116-123

[62] Tamirou T, Waeyenberg L, Tesfaye H, Ehlers R-U, Puza V, Mráček Z. *Steinernema ethiopiense* sp. n. (Rhabditida: Steinernematidae), a new entomopathogenic nematode from Ethiopia. Nematology. 2012;**14**:741-757 DOI: 10.1163/156854112X627282

[63] Mekete T, Gaugler R, Nguyen KB, Mandefro W, Tessera T. Biogeography of entomopathogenic nematodes in Ethyopia. Nematropica. 2005;**35**(1):31-35

[64] Waturu CN. Entomopathogenic nematodes (Steinernematidae and Heterorhabditidae) from Kenya [PhD Thesis]. Reading, UK: University of Reading; 1998

[65] Waturu CN, Hunt DJ, Reid AP. *Steinernema karii* sp. n. (Nematoda: Steinernematidae), a new entomopathogenic nematode from Kenya. International Journal of Nematology. 1997;**7**:65-75

[66] Mwaniki SW, Nderitu JH, Olubayo F, Nguyen K. Factors influencing the occurrence of entomopathogenic nematodes in the Central Rift Valley Region of Kenya. African Journal of Ecology. 2008;**46**:79-84. DOI: 10.1111/j.1365-2028.2008.00933.x

[67] Stack CM, Easwaramoorthy SG, Metha UK, Downes MJ, Griffin CT, Burnell AM. Molecular characterisation of *Heterorhabditis indica* isolates from India, Kenya, Indonesia and Cuba. Nematology. 2000;**2**(5):477-487. DOI: 10.1163/156854100509321

[68] Akalach M, Wright DJ. Control of the larvae of *Conorhynchus mendicus* (Col.: Curculionidae) by *Steinernema carpocapsae* and *Steinernema feltiae* (Nematoda: Steinernematidae) in the Gharb area (Morocco). Entomophaga. 1995;**40**(3-4):321-327. ISSN: 0013-8959

[69] Akyazi F, Ansari MA, Ahmed BI, Crow WT, Mekete T. First record of entomopathogenic nematodes (Steinernematidae and Heterorhabditidae) from Nigerian soil and their morphometrical and ribosomal DNA sequence analysis. Nematologia Mediterranea. 2012;**40**(2):95-100

[70] Yan X, Waweru B, Qiu X, Hategekimana A, Kajuga J, Li H, Edgington S, Umulisa S, Han R, Toepfer S. New entomopathogenic nematodes from semi-natural and small-holder farming habitats of Rwanda. Biocontrol Science and Technology. 2016;**26**(6):820-834 DOI: http://dx.doi.org/10.1080/09583157.2016.1159658

[71] Malan AP, Knoetze R, Moore SD. Isolation and identification of entomopathogenic nematodes from citrus orchards and their biocontrol potential against false codling moth. Journal of Invertebrate Pathology. 2011;**108**(2):115-125. DOI: 10.1016/j.jip.2011.07.006

[72] Hatting J, Stock SP, Hazir, S. Diversity and distribution of entomopathogenic nematodes (Steinernematidae, Heterorhabditidae) in South Africa. Journal of Invertebrate Pathology. 2009;**102**(2):120-128. DOI: 10.1016/j.jip.2009.07.003

[73] Malan AP, Nguyen KB, De Waal JY, Tiedt L. *Heterorhabditis safricana* n. sp. (Rhabditida : Heterorhabditidae), a new entomopathogenic nematode from South Africa. Nematology. 2008;**10**(3):381-396: DOI: 10.1163/156854108783900258

[74] Çimen H, Puza V, Nermut J, Hatting J, Ramakuwela T, Faktorova L, Hazir S. *Steinernema beitlechemi* n. sp., a new entomopathogenic nematode (Nematoda: Steinernematidae) from South Africa. Nematology. 2016;**18**:439-453. DOI: 10.1163/15685411-00002968

[75] Abate BA, Malan AP, Tiedt LR, Wingfield MJ, Slippers B, Hurley BP. *Steinernema fabii* n. sp. (Rhabditida: Steinernematidae), a new entomopathogenic nematode from South Africa. Nematology. 2016;**18**(2):235-255. DOI: 10.1163/15685411-00002956

[76] Çimen H, Lee MM, Hatting J, Hazir S, Stock SP. *Steinernema innovationi* n. sp (Panagrolaimomorpha: Steinernematidae), a new entomopathogenic nematode species from South Africa. Journal of Helminthology. 2015;**89**(4):415-427. DOI: https://doi.org/10.1017/S0022149X14000182

[77] Malan AP, Knoetze R, Tiedt L. Steinernema jeffreyense n. sp. (Rhabditida: Heterorhabditidae), a new entomopathogenic nematode from South Africa. Journal of Helminthology. 2015;**90**(3):262-278. DOI: https://doi.org/10.1017/S0022149X15000097.

[78] Nthenga I, Knoetze R, Berry S, Tiedt LR, Malan AP. *Steinernema sacchari* n. sp. (Rhabditida: Steinernematidae), a new entomopathogenic nematode from South Africa. Nematology. 2014;**16**(4):475-494. DOI: 10.1163/15685411-00002780

[79] Çimen H, Lee MM, Hatting J, Hazir S, Stock SP. *Steinernema tophus* sp n. (Nematoda: Steinernematidae), a new entomopathogenic nematode from South Africa. Zootaxa. 2014;**3821**(3):337-353. DOI: 10.11646/zootaxa.3821.3.3

[80] Malan AP, Knoetze R, Tiedt L. *Heterorhabditis noenieputensis* n. sp. (Rhabditida: Heterorhabditidae), a new entomopathogenic nematode from South Africa. Journal of Helminthology. 2014;88(2):139-151. DOI: https://doi.org/10.1017/S0022149X12000806

[81] Malan AP, Knoetze R, Tiedt L. *Steinernema nguyeni n* sp. (Rhabditida : Steinernematidae), a new entomopathogenic nematode from South Africa. Nematology. 2016; 18(5):571-590. DOI: 10.1163/15685411-00002978

[82] Půža V, Nermut J, Mráček Z, Gengler S. *Steinernema pwaniensis* n. sp., a new entomopathogenic nematode (Nematoda: Steinernematidae) from Tanzania. Journal of Helminthology. 2017;**91**(1):20-34. DOI: https://doi.org/10.1017/S0022149X15001157

[83] Gouge DH. Applications for social insect control. In: Grewal PS, Ehlers R-U, Shapiro-Ilan DI, editors. Nematodes as biocontrol agents. Wallingford, UK: CABI Publishing; 2005. pp. 317-329. DOI: 10.1079/9780851990170.0317

[84] Vashisth S, Chandel YS, Sharma PK. Entomopathogenic nematodes – A review. Agricultural Reviews. 2013;**34**(3):163-175. DOI: 10.5958/j.0976-0741.34.3.001

[85] Hazir S, Kaya HK, Stock, SP, Keskin N. Entomopathogenic nematodes (Steinernematidae and Heterorhabditidae) for biological control of soil pests. Turkish Journal of Biology. 2004;**27**:181-202. E-ISSN: 1303-6092, ISSN: 1300-1052

[86] Kaya HK, Gaugler R. Entomopathogenic nematodes. Annual Review of Entomology. 1993;**38**:181-206. DOI: 10.1146/annurev.en.38.010193.001145

[87] Kaya HK. Entomogenous and entomopathogenic nematodes in biological control. In: Evans K, Trudgill DL, Webster JM, editors. Plant Parasitic Nematodes in Temperate Agriculture. Wallingford, UK: CAB International; 1993. pp. 565-591. ISBN-13: 978-0851988085, ISBN-10: 0851988083

[88] Georgis R, Kaya HK. Formulation of entomopathogenic nematodes. In: Burges HD, editor. Formulation of Microbial Biopesticides: Beneficial Microorganisms, Nematodes and Seed Treatments. Dordrecht, The Netherlands: Kluwer; 1998. pp. 289-308. DOI: 10.1007/978-94-011-4926-6

[89] Rovesti L, Deseö KV. Compatibility of chemical pesticides with the entomopathogenic nematodes, *Steinernema carpocapsae* Weiser and *S. feltiae* Filipjev (Nematoda: Steinernematidae). Nematologica. 1990;**36**:237-245. DOI: 10.1163/002925990X00202

[90] Ishibashi N. Integrated control of insect pests by *Steinernema carpocapsae*. In: Bedding R, Akhurst R, Kaya HK, editors. Nematodes and the Biological Control of Insects. East Melbourne, Australia: CSRIO Publications; 1993. pp. 105-113. ISBN : 0643105913, 9780643105911

[91] Sinhouenon BG, Schiffers B, Baimey H, Wauters L, Dossou R, Ahissou R. Effet de quelques insecticides chimiques sur l'efficacité des nématodes entomopathogènes dans la lutte contre la teigne des crucifères: *Plutella xylostella* (L.) (Lépidoptères: Plutellidae) inféodés au chou à Djougou et à Ouaké, Bénin. In : 2e Colloque de l'Université de Parakou, du 23 au 25 Novembre 2015 sur le thème : La Recherche Scientifique au Service du Développement Local. Résumés des communications. Campus du Centre Universitaire de Parakou, Bénin. Programme des communications; 2015. p. 78. ISSN: 678-99919-62-55-9

[92] Stark JD. Entomopathogenic nematodes (Rhabditida: Steinernematidae): Toxicity of neem. Journal of Economic Entomology. 1996; **89**:68-73. DOI: 10.1093/jee/89.1.68

[93] Kaya HK, Burlando TM, Choo HY, Thurson GS. Integration of entomopathogenic nematodes with *Bacillus thuringiensis* or pesticidal soap for control of insect pests. Biological Control. 1995;**5**(3):432-441. DOI: 10.1006/bcon.1995.1052

[94] Sher RB, Parrella MP, Kaya HK. Biological control of the leafminer *Liriomyza trifolii* (Burgess): Implications for intraguild predation between *Diglyphus begini* Ashmead and *Steinernema carpocapsae* Weiser. Biological Control. 2000;**17**:155-163. DOI: 10.1006/bcon.1999.0794

[95] Koppenhöfer AM, Brown IM, Gaugler R, Grewal PS, Kaya HK, Klein MG. Synergism of entomopathogenic nematodes and imidacloprid against white grubs: Greenhouse and field evaluation. Biological Control. 2000;**19**(3):245-251. DOI: https://doi.org/10.1006/bcon.2000.0863

[96] Nishimatsu T, Jackson JJ. Interaction of insecticides, entomopathogenic nematodes, and larvae of the western corn rootworm (Coleoptera: Chrysomelidae). Journal of Economic Entomology. 1998;**91**(2):410-418. PMID: 9589627

[97] Thurston GS, Kaya HK, Gaugler R. Characterizing the enhanced susceptibility of milky disease-infected scarabaeid grubs to entomopathogenic nematodes. Biological Control. 1994;**4**(1):67-73. DOI: https://doi.org/10.1006/bcon.1994.1012

[98] Koppenhöfer AM, Choo HY, Kaya HK, Lee DW, Gelernter WD. Increased field and greenhouse efficacy against scarab grubs with a combination of an entomopathogenic nematode and *Bacillus thuringiensis*. Biological Control. 1999;**14**(1):37-44. DOI: 10.1006/bcon.1998.0663

[99] Ciche TA, Darby C, Ehlers R-U, Forst S, Goodrich-Blair H. Dangerous liaisons: the symbiosis of entomopathogenic nematodes and bacteria. Biological Control. 2006;**38**(1):22-46. DOI: https://doi.org/10.1016/j.biocontrol.2005.11.016

[100] Grewal PS. Formulation and application technology. In: Gaugler R, editor. Entomopathogenic Nematology. Wallingford, UK: CABI Publishing; 2002. pp. 265-287. ISBN: 0-85199-567-5

[101] Kowalska J. Entomopathogenic nematodes, insects, bacteria and their relationship used in practice. Wiadomości parazytologiczne. 2006;**52**(2):93-98. PMID: 17120989

[102] Barabara CA, Dowds BCA, Peters A. Virulence mechanisms. In: Gaugler R, editor. Entomopathogenic Nematology. Wallingford, UK: CABI Publishing; 2002. pp. 79-98. ISBN: 0-85199-567-5

[103] Zhou XS, Kaya HK, Heungens K, Goodrich-Blair H. Response of ants to a deterrent factor(s) produced by the symbiotic bacteria of entomopathogenic nematodes. Applied and Environmental Microbiology. 2002;**68**(12):6202-6209. DOI: 10.1128/AEM.68.12.6202.6209.2002

[104] Fenton A, Magoolagan L, Kennedy Z, Spencer KA. Parasite-induced warning coloration: A novel form of host manipulation. Animal Behaviour. 2011;**81**(2):417-422. DOI: 10.1016/j.anbehav.2010.11.010

[105] Koppenhofer AM, Fuzy EM. Soil moisture effects on infectivity and persistence of the entomopathogenic nematodes *Steinernema scarabaei, S. glaseri, Heterorhabditis zealandica,* and *H. bacteriophora*. Applied Soil Ecology. 2007;**35**:128-139. DOI: 10.1016/j.apsoil.2006.05.007

[106] Zadji L, Baimey H, Afouda L, Moens M, Decraemer W. Comparative susceptibility of *Macrotermes bellicosus* and *Trinervitermes occidentalis* (Isoptera: Termitidae) to entomopathogenic nematodes from Benin. Nematology. 2014;**16**(6):719-727. DOI: 10.1163/15685411-00002800

[107] Ferreira T, Malan AP. *Xenorhabdus* and *Photorhabdus* bacterial symbionts of the entomopathogenic nematodes *Steinernema* and *Heterorhabditis* and their *in vitro* liquid mass culture: A review. African Entomology. 2014;**22**(1):1-14. DOI: 10.4001/003.022.0115

[108] Ramarao N, Nielsen-Leroux C, Lereclus D. The insect *Galleria mellonella* as a powerful infection model to investigate bacterial pathogenesis. Journal of Visualized Experiments. 2012; 11:1-7. DOI: 10.3791/4392

[109] Zadji L, Baimey H, Afouda L, Moens M, Decraemer W. Effectiveness of different *Heterorhabditis* isolates from Southern Benin for biocontrol of subterranean termite, *Macrotermes bellicosus* (Isoptera: Macrotermitinae) in laboratory trials. Nematology. 2014;**16**:109-120. DOI: 10.1163/15685411-00002749

[110] Ma J, Chen SL, Moens M, Han RC, De Clercq P. Efficacy of entomopathogenic nematodes (Rhabditida: Steinernematidae and Heterorhabditidae) against the chive gnat, *Bradysia odoriphaga*. Journal of Pest Science. 2013;**86**(3):551-561. DOI: 10.1007/s10340-013-0497-7

[111] Grewal PS, Selvan S, Gaugler R. Thermal adaptation of entomopathogenic nematodes: niche breadth for infection, establishment, and reproduction. Journal of Thermal Biology. 1994;**19**(4):245-253 DOI: https://doi.org/10.1016/0306-4565(94)90047-7

[112] Andalo V, Santos V, Moreira GF, Moreira C, Freire M, Moino A. Movement of *Heterorhabditis amazonensis* and *Steinernema arenarium* in search of corn fall armyworm larvae in artificial conditions. Scientia Agricola. 2012;**69**:226-230. DOI: http://dx.doi.org/10.1590/S0103-90162012000300008

[113] Gulcu B, Hazir S, Kaya HK. Scavenger deterrent factor (SDF) from symbiotic bacteria of entomopathogenic nematodes. Journal of Invertebrate Pathology. 2012;**110**:326-333. DOI: 10.1016/j.jip.2012.03.014

[114] Ma J, Chen S, Moens M, De Clercq P, Li X, Han R. Characterization in biological traits of entomopathogenic nematodes isolated from North China. Journal of Invertebrate Pathology. 2013;**114**(3):268-276. DOI: 10.1016/j.jip.2013.08.012

[115] Shapiro-Ilan D, Brown I, Lewis EE. Freezing and desiccation tolerance in *Entomopathogenic* nematodes: Diversity and correlation of traits. Journal of Nematology. 2014;**46**(1):27-34. ISSN: 0022-300X

[116] Kung S, Gaugler R. Effects of soil temperature, moisture, and relative humidity on entomopathogenic nematode persistence. Journal of Invertebrate Pathology. 1991;**57**:242-249. ISSN: 0022-2011

[117] Morton A, Garcia-del-Pino F. Ecological characterization of entomopathogenic nematodes isolated in stonefruit orchard soils of Mediterranean areas. Journal of Invertebrate Pathology. 2009;**102**(3):203-213. DOI: 10.1016/j.jip.2009.08.002

[118] Perez EE, Lewis EE, Shapiro-Ilan DI. Impact of the host cadaver on survival and infectivity of entomopathogenic nematodes (Rhabditida: Steinernematidae and Heterorhabditidae) under desiccating conditions. Journal of Invertebrate Pathology. 2003;**82**(2):111-118. DOI: 10.1016/S0022-2011(02)00204-5

[119] Serwe-Rodriguez J, Sonnenberg K, Appleman B, Bornstein-Forst S. Effects of host desiccation on development, survival, and infectivity of entomopathogenic nematode *Steinernema carpocapsae*. Journal of Invertebrate Pathology. 2004;**85**(3):175-181. DOI: 10.1016/j.jip.2004.03.003

[120] Jagdale GB, Grewal PS. Acclimation of entomopathogenic nematodes to novel temperatures: Trehalose accumulation and the acquisition of thermotolerance. International Journal for Parasitology. 2003;**33**(2):145-152. DOI: 10.1016/S0020-7519(02)00257-6

[121] Shapiro-Ilan DI, Stuart RJ, McCoy CW. A comparison of entomopathogenic nematode longevity in soil under laboratory conditions. Journal of Nematology. 2006;**38**(1):119-129. ISSN: 0022-300X

[122] Ramakuwela T, Hatting H, Mark D, Laing MD, Hazir S, Thiebaut N. Effect of storage temperature and duration on survival and infectivity of *Steinernema innovationi* (Rhabditida: Steinernematidae). Journal of Nematology. 2015;**47**(4):332-336. PMCID: PMC4755708

[123] Jagdale GB, Grewal PS. Storage temperature influences desiccation and ultra violet radiation tolerance of entomopathogenic nematodes. Journal of Termal Biology. 2007;**32**(1):20-27. DOI: 10.1016/j.jtherbio.2006.07.004

[124] Hang TD, Choo HY, Lee DW, Lee SM, Kaya HK, Park CG. Temperature effects on Korean entomopathogenic nematodes, *Steinernema glaseri* and *S. longicaudum*, and their symbiotic bacteria. Journal of Microbiology Biotechnology. 2007;**17**(3):420-427. PMID: 18050945

[125] Kaya HK. Natural enemies and other antagonists. In: Gaugler R, editor. Entomopathogenic Nematology. New York: CABI; 2002. pp. 189-204. ISBN: 0-85199-567-5

[126] Shapiro D I, McCoy CW, Fares A, Obreza T, Dou H. Effects of soil type on virulence and persistence of entomopathogenic nematodes in relation to control of *Diaprepes abbreviatus*. Environmental Entomology. 2000;**29**(5):1083-1087. DOI: 10.1603/0046-225X-29.5.1083

[127] Millar LC, Barbercheck ME. Effects of tillage practices on entomopathogenic nematodes in a corn agroecosystem. Biological Control. 2002;**25**(1):1-11. DOI: 10.1016/S1049-9644(02)00042-7

[128] Grewal PS, Wang X, Taylor RAJ. Dauer juvenile longevity and stress tolerance in natural populations of entomopathogenic nematodes: Is there a relationship? International Journal for Parasitology. 2002;**32**(6):717-725. DOI: PMID: 12062490

[129] Adel MM, Hussein HM. Effectiveness of entomopathogenic nematodes *Steinernema feltiae* and *Heterorhabditis bacteriophora* on the Colorado potato beetle Leptinotarsa decemlineata (Say) (Coleoptera: Chrysomelidae) under laboratory and greenhouse conditions. Archives of Phytopathology and Plant Protection. 2010;**43**(15):1485-1494. DOI: 10.1080/03235400802538473

[130] Odendaal D, Addison MF, Malan AP. Evaluation of above-ground application of entomopathogenic nematodes for the control of diapausing codling moth (*Cydia pomonella* L.) under natural conditions. African Entomology. 2016;**24**(1):61-74. DOI: 10.4001/003.024.0061

[131] Campbell JF, Lewis EE, Stock SP, Nadler S, Kaya HK. Evolution of host search strategies in entomopathogenic nematodes. Journal of Nematology. 2003;**35**(2):142-145. PMC2620628

[132] Lacey LA, Georgis R. Entomopathogenic nematodes for control of insect pests above and below ground with comments on commercial production. Journal of Nematology. 2012;**44**(2):218-225. PMCID: PMC358470

[133] Cagnolo S, Campos V. Effect of storage temperature on survival and infectivity of *Steinernema rarum* (OLI strain) (Rhabditida: Steinernematidae). Journal of Invertebrate Pathology. 2008;**98**(1) :114-115. DOI:: 10.1016/j.jip.2008.02.013

[134] Shapiro-Ilan DI, Han R, Qiu X. Production of entomopathogenic nematodes. In: Morales-Ramos J, Rojas G, Shapiro-Ilan DI, editors. Mass Production of Beneficial Organisms: Invertebrates and Entomopathogens. San Diego, CA: Academic Press; 2014. pp. 321-356. ISBN-13: 978-0123914538, ISBN-10: 0123914531

[135] Solomon A, Salomon R, Paperna I, Glazer I. Desiccation stress of entomopathogenic nematodes induces the accumulation of a novel heat-stable protein. Parasitology. 2000;**121**:409-416. DOI: PMID: 11072904

[136] Grewal PS, Jagdale GB. Enhanced trehalose accumulation and desiccation survival of entomopathogenic nematodes through cold preacclimation. Biocontrol Science and Technology. 2002;**12**(5):533-545. DOI: 10.1080/0958315021000016207

[137] Molyneux AS. *Heterorhabditis* spp. and *Steinernema* spp. temperature and aspects of behaviour and infectivity. Experimental Parasitology. 1986;**62**(2):169-180. DOI: 10.1016/0014-4894(86)90021-4

[138] Kaya HK. Soil ecology. In: Gaugler R, Kaya HK, editors. Entomopathogenic Nematodes in Biological Control. Boca Raton, FL: CRC Press; 1990. pp. 93-116. ISBN: 0-8493-4541-3

[139] Shapiro-Ilan DI, Glazer I, Segal D. Trait stability and fitness of the heat tolerant entomopathogenic nematode *Heterorhabditis bacteriophora* IS5 strain. Biological Control. 1996;**6**(2):238-244 DOI: 10.1006/bcon.1996.0030

[140] Strauch O, Niemann I, Neumann A, Schmidt AJ, Peters A, Ehlers R-U. Storage and formulation of the entomopathogenic nematodes *Heterorhabditis indica* and *H. bacteriophora*. Biocontrol. 2000;**45**(4):483-500. DOI: 10.1023/A:1026528727365

[141] San-Blas E. Progress on entomopathogenic nematology research: A bibliometric study of the last three decades: 1980-2010. Biological Control. 2013;**66**:102-124. DOI: 10.1016/j.biocontrol.2013.04.002

[142] Grewal P, Georgis R. Entomopathogenic nematodes. In: Hall FR, Menn JJ, editors. Methods in Biotechnology. Vol. 5. Biopesticides: Use and delivery. Totowa, NJ: Humana Press; 1999. pp. 271-299. pISBN: 978-0-89603-515-7, eISBN: 978-1-59259-483-2

[143] Friedman MJ. Commercial production and development. In: Gaugler R, Kaya HK, editors. Entomopathogenic Nematodes in Biological Control. Boca Raton, FL: CRC Press; 1990. pp. 153-172. ISBN: 0-8493-4541-3

[144] Kaya HK, Stock SP. Techniques in insect nematology. In: Lacey L, editor. Manual of Techniques in Insect Pathology. San Diego, CA: Academic Press; 1997. pp. 281-324. eISBN: 9780123869005, pISBN: 9780123868992

[145] Gaugler R, Brown I, Shapiro-Ilan D, Atwa A. Automated technology for in vivo mass production of entomopathogenic nematodes. Biological Control. 2002;**24**(2):199-206. DOI: 10.1016/S1049-9644(02)00015-4

[146] Han RC, Ehlers R-U. Pathogenicity, development, and reproduction of *Heterorhabditis bacteriophora* and *Steinernema carpocapsae* under axenic *in vivo* conditions. Journal of Invertebrate Pathology. 2000;**75**(1):55-58. DOI: 10.1006/jipa.1999.4900

[147] Bai C, Shapiro-Ilan DI, Gaugler R, Hopper KR. Stabilization of beneficial traits in *Heterorhabditis bacteriophora* through creation of inbred lines. Biological Control. 2005;**32**(2):220-227. DOI: 10.1016/j.biocontrol.2004.09.011

[148] Ehlers R-U. Current and future use of nematodes in biocontrol: Practice and commercial aspects with regard to regulatory policy issues. Biocontrol Science and Technology. 1996;**6**(3):303-316. DOI: 10.1080/09583159631299

[149] Grewal PS, Georgis R. Entomopathogenic nematodes. In: Hall FR, Menn J, editors. Methods in Biotechnology, 5: Biopesticides: Use and Delivery. Humana Press. Totowa, NJ; 1998. pp. 271-299. ISBN-13: 978-0896035157, ISBN-10: 0896035158

[150] Ehlers R-U. Mass production of entomopathogenic nematodes for plant protection. Applied Microbiology and Biotechnology. 2001;**56**:523-633. DOI: PMID: 11601608

[151] Gaugler R, Han R. Production technology. In: Gaugler R, editor. Entomopathogenic Nematology. Wallingford, UK: CABI Publishing; 2002. pp. 289-320. ISBN: 0-85199-567-5

[152] Ehlers R-U. Achievements in research of EPN mass production. In: Griffin CT, Burnell AM, Downes MJ, editors. Developments in Entomopathogenic Nematode/Bacterial Research. Proceedings of the Workshop held at the National University of Ireland Maynooth, 13-15 April 2000. Luxemburg: European Union; 2001. pp. 68-77. ISBN: 92-894-0467-1

[153] Gaugler R, Grewal P, Kaya HK, Smith-Fiola D. Quality assessment of commercially produced entomopathogenic nematodes. Biological Control. 2000;**17**(1):100-109. DOI: 10.1006/bcon.1999.0768

[154] Goud S, Huger PS, Prabhuraj A. Effect of temperature, population density and shelf life of EPN *Heterorhabditis indica* (RCR) in sodium alginate gel formulation. Journal of Biopesticides. 2010;**3**(3):627-632

[155] Mejia-Torres MC, Saenz AA. Biological characterization of the Colombian isolate *Heterorhabditis so*. SL0708 (Rhabditida: Heterorhabditidae). Acta Scientiarum. 2013;**35**(3):445-449. DOI: 10.4025/actascibiolsci.v35i3.16034

[156] Grewal PS. Anhydrobiotic potential and long-term storage of entomopathogenic nematodes (Rhabditida: Steinernematidae). International Journal of Parasitology. 2000;**30**:995-1000. PMID: 10980289

[157] Navon A, Ascher KRS. Bioassays of Entomopathogenic Microbes and Nematodes. Wallingford, UK: CAB International; 2000. pp. 229-234. DOI: 10.1079/9780851994222.0000

[158] Merrill JH. Life-history and habits of two new nematodes parasitic on insects. Journal of Economic Entomology. 1916;**9**(1):148-149. DOI: 10.1093/jee/9.1.148

[159] Pemberton CE. Nematodes associated with termites in Hawaii, Borneo and Celebes. Proceedings of the Hawaiian Entomological Society; 1928. pp. 7:148-7:150. DOI: http://hdl.handle.net/10125/15760

[160] Tamashiro M. Susceptibility of Termites to Microbes. A Research Proposal submitted to the Office of Naval Research. Honolulu: Department of Entomology, University of Hawaii; 1968. p. 7

[161] Yu H, Gouge DH, Baker PB. Parasitism of subterranean termites (Isoptera: Rhinotermitidae) by entomopathogenic nematodes (Rhabditidae: Heterorhabditidae). Journal of Economic Entomology. 2006;**99**(4):1112-1119. PMID: 16937662

[162] Yu H, Gouge DH, Stock SP, Baker PB. Development of entomopathogenic nematodes (Rhabditida: Steinernematidae: Heterorhabditidae) in the desert subterranean termite Heterotermes aureus (Isoptera: Rhinotermitidae). Journal of Nematology. 2008;**40**(4):311-317. SN: 0022-300X

[163] Ibrahim SAM, El-Latif NA. A laboratory study to control subterranean termites. *Psammotermes hybostoma* (Desn.) (Isoptera: Rhinotermitidae) using entomopathogenic nematodes. Egyptian Journal of Biological Pest Control. 2008;**18**(1):99-103. ISSN: 1110-1768

[164] Shahina F, Tabassum KA, Salma J, Mahreen G. Biopesticidal affect of *Photorhabdus luminescens* against *Galleria mellonella* larvae and subterranean termite (Termitidae: Macrotermis). Pakistan Journal of Nematology 2011;**29**(1), 35-43. Available from: https://www.researchgate.net/publication/267959795

[165] Houesse AM. Evaluation du potential de quelques nematodes entomopathogènes du Bénin dans la lutte contre le charançon de la patate douce (*Cylas puncticollis* Boheman) en conditions de laboratoire. [Master Thesis]. Bénin: University of Parakou; 2017

[166] Abbott WS. A method of computing the effectiveness of an insecticide. Journal of Economic Entomology. 1925; **18**(2):265-267. DOI: https://doi.otg/10.1093/jee/18.2.265a

[167] Mauldin JK, Beal RH. Entomogenous nematodes for control of subterranean termites, *Reticulitermes* spp. Journal of Economic Entomology. 1989;**82**(6):1638-1642. DOI: 10.1093/jee/82.6.1638

[168] Gaugler R, Lewis E, Stuart RJ. Ecology in the service of biological control: The case of entomopathogenic nematodes. Oecologia. 1997;**109**(4):483-489. DOI: 10.1007/s0074420050108

[169] Wilson-Rich N, Stuart RJ, Rosengaus RB. Susceptibility and behavioral response of the dampwood termite *Zootermopsis angusticollis* to the entomopathogenic nematode *Steinernema carpocapsae*. Journal of Invertebrate Pathology. 2007;**95**:17-25. DOI: 10.1016/j.jip.2006.11.004

[170] Georgis R, Dunlop DB, Grewal PS. Formulation of entomopathogenic nematodes. In: Hall FR, Barry JW, editors. Biorational Pest Control Agents: Formulation and Delivery. ACS Symposium Series No. 595. Washington, D.C.: American Chemical Society; 1995. pp. 197-205. ISBN: 0841232261

[171] Lenz M, Runko S. Potential of Two Microbial Pathogens for the Management of Infestations of *Neotermes* sp. in Crop Trees on Rotuma, Fiji. Commonwealth Scientific and Industrial Research Organization, Division of Entomology. Termite Group Report No. 95/4; 1995. p. 60

[172] Lenz M, Kamath MK, Lal S, Senivasa E. Status of the Tree Damaging *Neotermes sp.* in Fiji's American Mahogany Plantation and Preliminary Evaluation of the Use of Entomopathogens for Their Control. Project Report, ACIAR Small Project No. FST/96/205; 2000. p. 111

[173] Susurluk A., Ehlers R-U. Field persistence of the entomopathogenic nematode *Heterorhabditis bacteriophora* in different crops. BioControl. 2008;**53**(4):627-641. DOI: 10.1007/s10526-007-9104-2

[174] Epsky ND, Capinera JL. Efficacy of the entomogenous nematode *Steinernema feltiae* against a subterranean termite, *Reticulitermes tibialis* (Isoptera: Rhinotermitidae). Journal of Economic Entomology. 1988;**81**(5):1313-1317. DOI: 10.1093/jee/81.5.1313

[175] Gaugler R, Wang Y, Campbell JF. Aggressive and evasive behaviors in *Popillia japonica* (Coleoptera: Scarabaeidae) larvae: Defenses against entomopathogenic nematode attack. Journal of Invertebrate Pathology. 1994;**64**(3):193-199. DOI: 10.1016/S0022-2011(94)90150-3

[176] Koppenhöfer AM, Grewal PS, Kaya HK. Synergism of imidacloprid and entomopathogenic nematodes against white grubs: The mechanism. Entomologia Experimentalis et Applicata. 2000;**94**(3):283-293. DOI: 10.1046/j.1570-7458.2000.00630.x

[177] Mankowski M, Kaya HK, Grace JK, Sipes BS. Differential susceptibility of subterranean termite castes to entomopathogenic nematodes. Biocontrol Science and Technology. 2005;**15**(4):367-377. DOI: 10.1080/09583150400016951

[178] Fujii JK. Effects of an entomogenous nematode *Neoaplectana carpocapsae* Weiser, on the Formosan subterranean termite, *Coptotermes formosanus* [Ph.D thesis]. University of Hawaii, Honolulu; 1975

[179] Woodrow RJ, Grace JK, Oshiro RJ. Comparison of localized injections of spinosad and selected insecticides for the control of *Cryptotermes brevis* (Isoptera: Kalotermitidae) in naturally infested structural mesocosms. Journal of Economic Entomology. 2006;**99**(4):1354-1362. PMID: 16937692

[180] Grace JK, Woodrow RJ, Oshiro RJ. Expansive gallery systems of one-piece termites (Isoptera: Kalotermitidae). Sociobiology. 2009;**54**(1):37-44. ISSN: 0361-6525

[181] Guirado N, Ambrosano EJ, Rossi F, Dias FLF. Controle de Cupins de Montículo com *Metarhizium anisopliae* e *Beauveria bassiana*. Revista Brasileira de Agroecologia. 2009;**4**(2):23-26 (in Portuguese). ISSN : 1980-9735

[182] Toscano LC, Schlick-Souza EC, Martins GLM, Souza-Schlick GD, Maruyama WT. Controle do cupim de montículo (Isoptera: Termitidae) de pastagem com fungos entomopatogênicos. Revista Caatinga. 2010;**23**(2):6-11 (in Portuguese). pISSN: 0100-316X, eISSN: 1983-2125

[183] Boucias DG, Stokes C, Storey G, Pendland JC. The effect of imidacloprid on the termite *Reticulitermes flavipes* and its interaction with the mycopathogen *Beauveria bassiana*. Pfanzenschutz-Nachr. Bayer 1996;**49**:103-145

[184] Ramakrishnan R, Suiter DR, Nakatsu CH, Humber RA. Imidacloprid-enhanced *Reticulitermes flavipes* (Isoptera: Rhinotermitidae) susceptibility to the entomopathogen *Metarhizium anisopliae*. Journal of Economic Entomology. 1999;**92**(5):1125-1132. DOI: 10.1093/jee/92.5.1125

[185] Su N-Y. Response of the Formosan subterranean termites (Isoptera: Rhinotermitidae) to baits or nonrepellent termiticides in extended foraging arenas. Journal of Economic Entomology. 2005;**98**:2143-2152. DOI: 10.1603/0022-0493-98.6.2143

Evolutionary Expansion of Nematode-Specific Glycine-Rich Secreted Peptides

Muying Ying, Mingyue Ren, Chenglin Liu and
Ping Zhao

Additional information is available at the end of the chapter

http://dx.doi.org/10.5772/intechopen.68621

Abstract

A genome-wide survey across 10 species from algae *Guillardia theta* to mammals revealed that *Caenorhabditis elegans* and *Caenorhabditis briggsae* acquired a large number of glycine-rich secreted peptides (GRSPs, 110 GRSPs in *C. elegans* and 93 in *C. briggsae*) during evolution in this study. Chromosomal mapping indicated that most GRSPs were clustered on their genomes [103 (93.64%) in *C. elegans* and 82 (88.17%) in *C. briggsae*]. Totally, there are 18 GRSPs cluster units in *C. elegans* and 13 in *C. briggsae*. Except for four *C. elegans* where GRSP clusters lacking matching clusters in *C. briggsae*, all other GRSP clusters had its corresponding orthologous clusters between the two nematodes. Using eight transcriptomic datasets of Affmyetrix microarray, genome-wide association studies identified many co-expressed GRSPs clusters after *C. elegans* infections. Highly homologous coding sequences and conserved exon-intron organizations indicated that GRSP tight clusters might have originated from local DNA duplications. The conserved synteny blocks of GRSP clusters between their genomes, the co-expressed GRSPs clusters after *C. elegans* infections, and a strong purifying selection of protein-coding sequences suggested evolutionary constraint acting on *C. elegans* to ensure that *C. elegans* could rapidly launch and fulfill systematic responses against infections by co-expression, co-regulation, and co-functionality of GRSP clusters.

Keywords: glycine-rich secreted peptide, synteny block, co-expressed gene cluster, nematode infection

1. Introduction

According to the primary structure, glycine-rich proteins can be classified into two classes: (1) consisting of large glycine-rich proteins (GRPs >200 AA) with a length of over 200 amino acids that typically function as cell wall structural components and (2) composed of small glycine-rich secreted peptides (GRSPs, <200 AA) that have a typical signal peptide followed by a mature peptide with a high glycine content. GRSPs represent a class of unique effectors of multicellular organisms, possessing relatively simple structures but exhibiting complex biological functions. According to previous research, almost all animals, plants, and microorganisms are enriched with GRPs, such as glycine-rich cold-induced proteins from zebrafish [1], glycine-rich keratin and keratin-associated proteins from 22 mammal genomes [2] and RNA-binding proteins with C-terminal glycine-rich domain from *Arabidopsis thaliana* [3]. Plant GRPs have shown diverse functions, including cell wall structure, plant defense, oleosin GRPs in pollen hydration and competition, extracellular ligands of kinase proteins, and RNA-binding GRPs in osmotic stress and cold stress [4]. Growing evidence suggests that these proteins play key roles in the adaptation of organisms to biotic and abiotic stresses including those resulting from pathogenesis, alterations in the osmotic, saline, and oxidative environment, and changes in temperature [3].

To our knowledge, total GRSPs encoded by genomes of different species are significantly distinct. GRSPs are enriched in some species, whereas in other species, no GRSPs have been identified. *Caenorhabditis elegans* and *Caenorhabditis briggsae* are highly enriched for GRSPs in this study. With relatively simple structures but complex biological functions, the importance of GRSPs in nematodes is highlighted by the observations that many members in the GRSP family were indicated to play important roles in *C. elegans* innate immunity. For example, *nlp-29* and *cnc-2* in the GRSP family were upregulated after *Serratia marcescens* infection of *C. elegans* [5]. *Nlp-29* and *nlp-31* in GRSP family were differentially expressed in response to fungal and bacterial infection [6]. Six members in GRSP family from *nlp-27* to *nlp-31* and *grsp-2* were upregulated after *Drechmeria coniospora* infection of *C. elegans* in vivo [7]. Expression of the family member *grsp-21* was upregulated twofold in response to *Microbacterium nematophilum* [8]. Evolutionary diversification of these GRSPs may enhance anti-fungal innate immunity of *C. elegans* [7]. Although these GRSPs are important for *C. elegans* innate immunity, we could not find its corresponding orthologs in human genome. As soil organisms and bacterial feeders, nematodes were constantly challenged by all the different species of soil bacteria, fungi, and other microbes, which have been driving the evolution of nematodes. We were impressed by published works about members of the GRSP family in immune responses of *C. elegans* and interested in knowing whether there were more GRSPs in nematodes and how GRSPs responded to *C. elegans* infections. We believed that free-living soil nematodes very likely to have developed unique components to adapt to the unique environment.

The importance of GRSP family in nematodes is further stressed by the fact that expression of certain GRSPs of *C. elegans* was upregulated by Gram−, Gram+, and fungi of natural infection. Supported by the above facts, we believed in the existence of additional GRSPs and hypothesized that analyzing the genomic sequence would identify novel GRSPs and provide a new global view of GRSP evolution in nematodes. To have a general knowledge of the two nematodes, in the present work, we particularly focused on (1) genome-wide identification and classification of GRSPs which would provide a global view of GRSPs evolution in the two nematodes, (2) mapping these GRSPs on their genomes which would provide a global view of GRSPs distributions on their chromosomes, (3) phylogenetic analyses based on signal peptides of the two nematode GRSPs, and (4) integrated analysis of public transcriptome datasets about *C. elegans* infections would gain insights into the role of *C. elegans* GRSPs in innate immune.

2. Materials and methods

2.1. Identification of GRSPs in the two nematode genomes

Comprehensive comparison of GRSPs was conducted across 10 species of genomes: *Homo sapiens, Danio rerio, Drosophila melanogaster, C. elegans, C. briggsae, A. thaliana, Monosiga brevicollis, Saccharomyces cerevisiae, Dictyostelium discoideum,* and *G. theta*. Genome-wide protein sequences of the 10 species were downloaded from the UCSC database (https://genome.ucsc.edu/), and it used to construct two local protein sequence databases. Local-Blastp and PSI-Blast programs from NCBI were carried out to identify *C. elegans* GRSPs with the previously identified GRSPs: *nlp-29, nlp-31, nlp-33, cnc-2, cnc-4,* and *cnc-6* as initial queries. GRSPs of *C. briggsae* were identified by using all *C. elegans* GRSPs as initiation queries.

2.2. *C. elegans* GRSPs expression at transcriptional level

Gene expression omnibus (GEO) data sets in NCBI (http://www.ncbi.nlm.nih.gov/) and the reads of RNA sequencing project (PRJNA33023) in DRASearch (https://trace.ddbj.nig.ac.jp/DRASearch/) were used to confirm the transcriptional expression of *C. elegans* GRSPs and avoid false positive arising from genome annotation. This RNA sequencing project is a component of the *C. elegans* modENCODE project including 308 SRA experiments and 196 Biosamples. The total number of genes on each chromosome of *C. elegans* was obtained from UCSC (WS220/ce10) for the estimate of GRSPs density on each chromosome.

2.3. Mapping GRSPs to the genomes of the two nematodes

Characteristic parameters of GRSPs were obtained from WormBase (https://www.wormbase.org/). Configuration files were generated, and mapping of GRSPs to the genomes was performed by Circos [9]. Spacing was based on chromosomal units and the results were further manually modified for easier identification. Orthologous pairs were determined by the twoway reciprocal "best hits" and combining sequence similarity- and synteny-based approaches. Orthologous GRSPs pairs were mapped to their genomes and connected across their chromosomal maps by straight line to identify conserved orthologous synteny blocks of the two nematode genomes.

2.4. Transcriptomic analysis of *C. elegans* GRSPs following infection

Eight transcriptomic data sets related to *C. elegans* infections quantified by Affymetrix microarray (GSE20053, E-MEXP-696, GSE27867, GSE54212, GSE53732, GSE41058, GSE37266, and GSE2740) were downloaded from NCBI GEO database. Differentially expressed GRSPs were extracted to analyze using the GEO2R tool in the GEO database. The range of co-expression clusters of *C. elegans* GRSPs was defined to be less than 500 kb. Due to the limited data sets of *C. briggsae* genome, we failed to confirm transcriptional expression of *C. briggsae* GRSPs to estimate GRSPs density on its chromosomes and to analyze the co-expressed *C. briggsae* GRSPs after infections.

2.5. Phylogenetic and evolutionary analysis

With the signal peptide sequences of the two nematode GRSPs, a phylogenetic tree was built to detect how the nematode GRSPs families had evolved by gene duplication by using the program Molecular Evolutionary Genetics Analysis package version 6 (MEGA 6) [10]. The bootstrap consensus tree inferred from 500 replicates was taken to represent the evolutionary history to assess the reliability of the phylogenetic tree using the neighbor-joining (NJ) method under p distance [11]. All sites bearing alignment gaps and missing information were retained initially, excluding them as necessary using the pairwise deletion option.

2.6. Analysis of the nucleotide sequences

Using MEGA 6, we estimated transition (Ti)/transversion (Tv) ratios (R) among nucleotides, the number of synonymous (dS) and nonsynonymous (dN) substitutions per site, and the codon-based Z-test for purifying selection. The program was operated under the model of the modified Nei-Gojobori (assumed Ti/Tv bias = 2,2) methods to calculate the difference of dN-dS, and the values were estimated by standard errors (SE) by the bootstrap methods (800 replicates; seed = 17,114) (for details, please refer to supplementary materials and methods in [12]).

3. Results

3.1. Genome-wide analysis of GRSPs across 10 species

The number of GRSPs in each genome of the 10 species was 4 for human, 6 for zebrafish, 53 for fruit fly, 110 for *C. elegans*, 93 for *C. briggsae*, 52 for *A. thaliana*, 0 for *M. brevicollis*, 0 for *S. cerevisiae*, 5 for *D. discoideum*, and 0 for *G.theta*. The two nematodes (110 for *C. elegans* and 93 for *C. briggsae*) are extremely enriched with GRSPs in this study. Analysis of *C. elegans* GRSPs in these species revealed that the number of twoway reciprocal "best hit" orthologs was respectively 0, 2, 8, 90, 3, 0, 0, 2, and 0 (**Table 1**) [12]. Few matching orthologs of *C. elegans* GRSPs in the other species may indicate that GRSPs were less vertically inherited. Besides the two nematodes, *D. melanogaster* and *A. thaliana* are also enriched for GRSPs when compared to the other species analyzed here, which may indicate that an evolutionary expansion of GRSPs happened in nematodes, arthropods, and plants over evolutionary adaption and speciation.

3.2. Identification and classification of the two nematode GRSPs

Based on sequence similarity and the conservation of intron position and phase, 203 GRSPs of the two nematodes were classified into 17 subfamilies (for details, please refer to Figure S1

Species name	Genome size (Mb)	Ref seq protein	Reference Bioproject	GRSPs	Orthologs of *C. elegans*
H. sapiens	3200	55968	PRJNA168	4	0
D. rerio	1371	47861	PRJNA13922	6	2
D. melanogaster	144	30275	PRJNA164	53	8
C. elegans	100	26047	PRJNA158	110	110
C. briggsae	104	17682	PRJNA20855	93	92
A. thaliana	120	35378	PRJNA116	52	3
M. brevicollis	42	9203	PRJNA28133	0	0
S. cerevisiae	12	5907	PRJNA128	0	0
D. discoideum	34	13315	PRJNA13925	5	2
G. theta	0.67	632	PRJNA210	0	0

Table 1. An estimated number of GRSPs in different species and the number of corresponding orthologs in *C. elegans*.

and S2 in [12]). GRSPs mature peptides are enriched for glycine with content ranging from 17 to 74% (For details, please refer to Table S3 in [12]). 62 GRSPs (30.54%) with glycine content from 30 to 40% are the most abundant (**Figure 1**). Among 110 *C. elegans* GRSPs, 36, 11, 14, and 2 have already been designated as "fungus-induced protein related" (FIPR) or "fungus-induced protein" (FIP), "*Caenorhabditis bacteriocin*" (CNC), "neuropeptide-like protein" (NLP), and "DAF-16/FOXO Controlled, germline Tumor affecting" (DCT) in public database. Based on

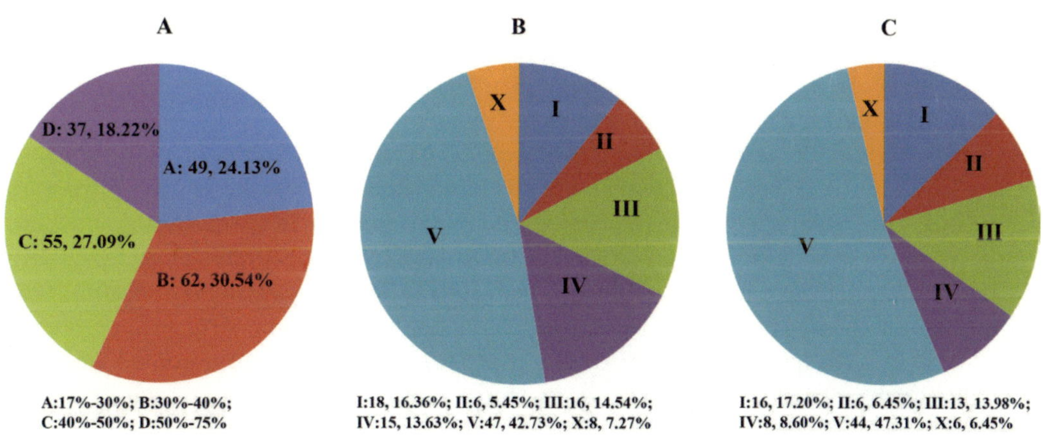

Figure 1. Statistic description of *C. elegans* and *C. briggsae* GRSPs. (A) The number of mature GRSPs peptides with different glycine contents: the number of mature GRSPs peptides with glycine content ranging from 17 to 30% is 49 (24.13%), from 30 to 40% is 62 (30.54%), from 40 to 50% is 55 (27.09%), and from 50 to 75% is 37 (18.23%). (B) The number and percentage of *C. elegans* GRSPs distributed on chromosomes: 18 (16.67%) GRSPs were found on chromosome I, 6 (5.45%) on chromosome II, 16 (14.54%) on chromosome III, 15 (13.63%) on chromosome IV, 47 (42.73%) on chromosome V, and 8 (7.27%) on chromosome X. (C) The number and percentage of *C. briggsae* GRSPs distributed on chromosomes: 16 (17.20%) GRSPs are found on chromosome I, 6 (6.45%) on chromosome II, 13 (13.98%) on chromosome III, 8 (8.60%) on chromosome IV, 44 (47.31%) on chromosome V, and 6 (6.45%) on chromosome X. Comparing S1B to S1C showed that the distribution ratio of GRSPs on its corresponding chromosomes of the two nematodes is similar.

the following shared characteristics: (1) a typical signal peptide located at the N-terminus, (2) a precursor peptide with less than 200 AA, (3) a predicted mature peptide with high glycine contents, and (4) by comparison with the three members (NP_001024238, NP_501117, and NP_504970) already named as GRSPs (*grsp-1*, *grsp-3*, and *grsp-4* in public database), we designated the other 47 unnamed peptides as GRSPs by these criteria. GRSPs identified in *C. briggsae* were referred to as "Cbr," representing the first three letters of the species name *C. briggsae*, plus the name of the corresponding orthologs in *C. elegans* following the previous study [7]. Except for *Cbr-grsp-32*, all the other *C. briggsae* GRSPs have its corresponding orthologs in *C. elegans*. The number of FIPR or FIP, CNC, NLP, and GRSPs family members in *C. briggsae* is, respectively, 31, 9, 12, and 41 (for details, please refer to Table S1 in [12]).

3.3. The evidence of transcriptional expression of *C. elegans* GRSPs

Highly homologous GRSPs are usually clustered together on the two nematode genomes. This is exemplified by GRSPs from *fipr-3* to *fipr-9* clustered on *C. elegans* chromosome V. Their percent identity of protein-coding sequence ranges from 86.1 to 100% (for details, please refer to Figure S4 in [12]). It is notorious that many short genes enriched for repeat sequences are frequently incorrect in genome annotation. To avoid false positive resulting from genome annotation, we further verified the transcriptional expression of all *C. elegans* GRSPs using the available public database. Evidence of transcriptional expression in GEO database showed that 65 *C. elegans* GRSPs were transcriptional expressions (for details, please refer to Table S1 in [12]). For the other 45 GRSPs without transcriptional evidence in GEO database, RNA reads from *C. elegans* transcriptome project were used to confirm their transcriptions, which showed that all GRSPs except for *fipr-12* had 100% matching reads in this project (for details, please refer to Figure S5 in [12]).

3.4. The clustered distribution of GRSPs on the two nematode genomes

GRSPs distribution on their genomes was marked by following qualities (**Figure 2** and **Table 2**): first, most of the GRSPs were clustered on their genomes. The criteria for the definition of GRSPs clusters are (1) the scale between closely adjacent GRSPs should be less than 1 Mb, (2) the number of GRSPs members are equal to or above 3, and (3) the scale of GRSPs clusters is less than 3 Mb. The number of GRSPs clustered on their genomes was 103 for *C. elegans* and 82 for *C. briggsae*. The number of GRSPs clusters is 18 for *C. elegans* and 13 for *C. briggsae*. Second, almost half of the GRSPs in the two nematodes were mapped on their chromosome V (47 in *C. elegans* and 44 in *C. briggsae*). The biggest cluster (from *fip-2* to *nlp-24*) on *C. elegans* chromosome V possesses 15 GRSPs. Of the total 3603 genes on *C. elegans* chromosome V, 47 GRSPs account for 1.30%.

Third, GRSPs clusters were maintained in relative conserved synteny blocks on the chromosomes of the two nematodes (**Figure 2** and **Table 2**). With the exception of four GRSPs clusters without the matching synteny clusters on *C. briggsae* genome, all the other GRSPs clusters possess the matching synteny clusters between the two nematodes. Generally, the lack of the four matching GRSPs synteny clusters in *C. briggsae* could be attributed to the following reasons: (1) no orthologs of *C. elegans* GRSPs were available in *C. briggsae*, (2) the orthologs of *C. elegans* GRSPs in *C. briggsae* were integrated into another unequal GRSPs cluster of *C. briggsae*, and (3) the map position of orthologs of *C. elegans* GRSPs on *C. briggsae* genome was changed. Some of the orthologous

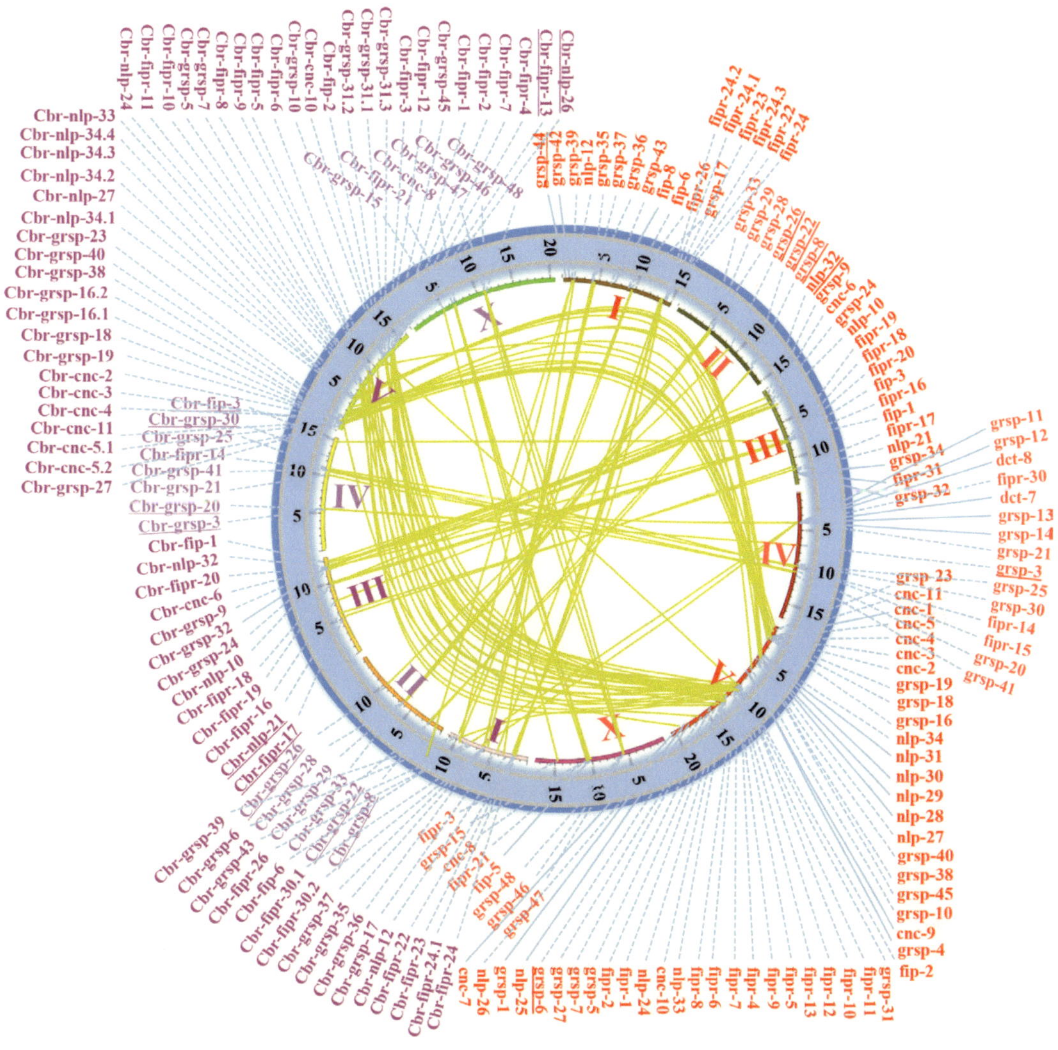

Figure 2. Mapping of GRSPs to genomes of the two nematodes is shown. *C.elegans* and *C. briggsae* GRSPs are indicated by red and purple letters, respectively, which are linked with their chromosomal location by a blue line. Letters from I-X represent chromosome serial numbers of *C. elegans* (red) and *C. briggsae* (purple). GRSPs orthologs between *C.elegans* and *C. briggsae* are linked by yellow beelines. GRSPs lacking orthologs between the two nematodes are linked by a blue solid line with their chromosomal location for easier identification. 7 *C. elegans* GRSPs (*grsp-44* on ChrI, *grsp-26*, *grsp-22*, and *grsp-8* on ChrII, *nlp-32* on ChrIII, *grsp-3* on ChrIV, and *grsp-6* on ChrV) and 11 *C. briggsae* GRSPs (*Cbr-grsp-26*, *Cbr-grsp-22* and *Cbr-grsp-8* on ChrII, *Cbr-fipr-17* and *Cbr-nlp-21* on ChrIII, *Cbr-grsp-3*, *Cbr-grsp-20*, *Cbr-grsp-30*, and *Cbr-fip-3* on ChrIV, *Cbr-fipr-13* and *Cbr-nlp-26* on ChrV) alone scattered on their respective genomes are indicated by an underline.

synteny clusters were observed one-to-two match on their genomes. For example, GRSPs cluster from *Cbr-grsp-27* to *Cbr-grsp-23* on *C. briggsae* chromosome V was matched to two orthologous synteny clusters (from *grsp-23* to *grsp-16* and from *grsp-40* to *grsp-4*) on *C. elegans* chromosome V.

In addition, the order of the orthologous synteny blocks of GRSPs clusters on chromosome V was more conserved than that on other chromosomes of the two nematodes. Orthologous pairs of GRSPs

Chromosome	Size(Mbp)		GRSPs/Gene	GRSPs cluster/ Scale	
	C. elegans	*C. briggsae*		*C. elegans*	*C. briggsae*
I	15.07	15.46	18/3807	From *grsp-42* to *nlp-12*/3GRSPs /904.87kb	From *Cbr-fipr-24* to *Cbr-nlp-12*/5GRSPs /563.98kb
				From *grsp-35* to *grsp-36*/3GRSPs /5.71kb	From *Cbr-grsp-17* to *Cbr-fipr-30.1*/6GRSPs /2.04Mb
				From *grsp43* to *grsp-17*/5GRSPs /2.53Mb	From *Cbr-fip-6* to *Cbr- grsp-39*/5GRSPs / 2.52Mb
				From *fipr-24.2* to *fipr-24*/6GRSPs / 6.6kb	
II	15.28	16.63	6/2648	From *grsp-33* to *grsp-28*/3GRSPs /1.7kb	From *Cbr-grsp-33* to *Cbr-grsp-28*/3GRSPs / 2.7kb
III	13.78	14.58	16/3665	From *grsp-9* to *nlp-10*/4GRSPs /2.17Mb	From *Cbr-fipr-16* to *Cbr-fipr-18*/3GRSPs /2.09Mb
				From *fipr-19* to *fip-1*/6GRSPs /1.18Mb	From *Cbr-nlp-10* to *Cbr-fip-1*/8GRSPs /1.19Mb
				From *fipr-17* to *grsp-32*/5GRSPs /802.9kb	
IV	17.49	17.49	15/3393	From *grsp-11* to *grsp-21*/8GRSPs /401.7kb	From *Cbr- grsp-21* to *Cbr-grsp-25*/4GRSPs /1.39Mb
				From *grsp-25* to *grsp-41*/6GRSPs /2.45Mb	
V	20.92	19.5	47/3603	From *grsp-23* to *grsp-16*/10GRSPs/781.2kb	From *Cbr-grsp-27* to *Cbr-grsp-23*/14GRSPs/ 1.52Mb
				From *nlp-34* to *nlp-27*/6GRSPs/10.3kb	From *Cbr-nlp-34.1* to *Cbr-nlp-34.4*/5GRSPs / 28.97kb
				From *grsp-40* to *grsp-4*/6GRSPs/2.71Mb	
				From *fip-2* to *nlp-24*/15GRSPs /2.54Mb	From *Cbr-nlp-33* to *Cbr-fipr-6*/10GRSPs /2.81Mb
				From *fipr-1* to *grsp-27*/5GRSPs/1.22Mb	From *Cbr-grsp-10* to *Cbr-fipr-4*/13GRSPs /1.78Mb
				From *nlp-25* to *cnc-7*/4GRSPs/786.58kb	
X	17.72	21.54	8/4818	From *grsp-47* to *grsp-48*/3GRSPs/3.16kb	From *Cbr-grsp-15* to *Cbr-cnc-8*/3GRSPs/2.22Mb
				From *fip-5* to *grsp-15*/5GRSPs/1.34Mb	From *Cbr-grsp-47* to *Cbr-grsp-48*/3GRSPs/3.08kb
Total	100.26	105.2	110/21932	18 cluster	13 cluster

Notes: Chr: Chromosome; Size: Chromosome size. GRSPs/Genes: GRSPs number/ total number of genes on each chromosome of *C. elegans*. GRSPs cluster/Scale, GRSPs in each cluster/ scale of GRSP clusters on chromosomes. Matching synteny clusters between the two nematodes were linked by dot lines. The criteria for the definition of GRSP clusters are: 1) distance between closely adjacent GRSPs is less than 1Mb; 2) GRSPs members are greater than or equal to 3; 3) scale of GRSP clusters is less than 3Mb.

Table 2. Summary of GRSPs clusters on the chromosomes of the two nematodes.

between the two nematodes were linked by straight lines on their genome mapping, which showed that the beelines of the orthologous GRSPs clusters on chromosomes V were more likely to be crossovers than those on other chromosomes (**Figure 2**). The crossover means that the order of orthologous synteny blocks of GRSPs clusters was maintained on the genomes of the two nematodes.

3.5. The transcriptional co-expression of *C. elegans* GRSPs clusters after infection

Genome-wide transcriptional analysis showed that many *C. elegans* genes that responded to infection were located in small genomic clusters [8]. All members of the GRSPs cluster from *nlp-27* to *nlp-34* were induced by *D. coniospora* infection of *C. elegans* [7]. Using the transcriptome data sets of *C. elegans* infection based on microarray quantification [7, 8, 13–16], we analyzed the transcriptional expression change of *C. elegans* GRSPs after *C. elegans* infection. The results showed that a total of 108 *C. elegans* GRSPs showed differential expressions at transcriptional levels after *C. elegans* infection in previous studies, which are indicated by blue letters in **Figure 3**. Co-expressed clusters of *C. elegans* GRSPs are shadowed by grey (**Table 3**)

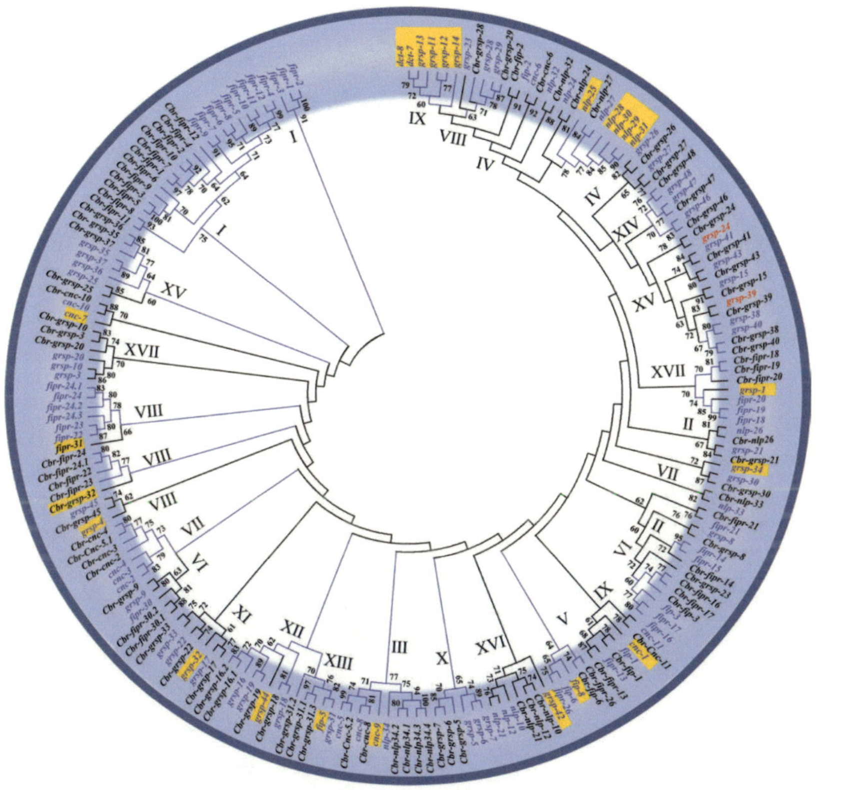

Figure 3. Phylogenetic analysis based on the typical signal peptides of GRSPs in *C. elegans* and *C. briggsae* is shown. The number from I-XVII represents different subfamilies. 24 GRSPs (23 *C. elegans* GRSPs and 1 *C. briggsae* GRSPs) lacking orthologs between the two nematodes are shadowed by orange color for easy identification. 108 of the 110 *C. elegans* GRSPs that had transcriptional expression after infection in previous studies are indicated by blue letters. Two *C. elegans* GRSPs (*grsp-24* and *grsp-39*) without detectable expression data in previous studies analyzed here are indicated by red letters.

Gene Name	Pathogenic	Reference
fip-8 fip-6; cnc-6 fip-3 fip-1; dct-7 grsp-21 (4.64kb) grsp-3 grsp-25; cnc-4 cnc-3 cnc-2 (2.53kb) nlp-34 nlp-31 nlp-30 nlp-29 (5.54kb) grsp-38 grsp-10 fip-2 fipr-11 nlp-33 nlp-24 cnc-7; grsp-46 fip-5 fipr-21 (1.79kb) grsp-15	*D. coniospora*	Pujol et al., 2008
grsp-4 grsp-42 nlp-12 grsp-35 grsp-37 grsp-36 (5.13kb) grsp-43 fipr-26 fipr-23 fipr-22 fipr-24 (4.35kb); grsp-8 grsp-26; nlp-32 nlp-10 fip-3 fipr-16 fip-1 (50.45kb) nlp-21 fipr-30 dct-7 grsp-13 grsp-21(20.91kb) grsp-3 grsp-41 grsp-25 grsp-23 grsp-45 grsp-40 grsp-38 (1.05kb) cnc-1 cnc-5 cnc-4 cnc-3 cnc-2 (5.75kb) grsp-19 grsp-18 grsp-16 (8.41kb) nlp-31 nlp-30 nlp-29 nlp-28 nlp-27 (9.24kb) grsp-10 fip-2 grsp-31(57.64kb) nlp-33 fipr-2 grsp-7 (38.69kb) grsp-27 nlp-26 cnc-7 grsp-46 grsp-47 fip-5 fipr-21 cnc-8 (3.88kb) grsp-15	*M. nematophilum*	O'Rourke et al., 2006
grsp-44 grsp-42 nlp-12 grsp-35 grsp-37 grsp-36 (5.13kb) grsp-43; grsp-41; nlp-30 grsp-40 grsp-38 (1.05kb) grsp-45 nlp-33 grsp-5 grsp-7 (1.48kb)	*P. aeruginosa*	Sun et al., 2011
fipr-22 fipr-23 (2.19kb) cnc-7 cnc-4	*C.albicans*	Pukkila-Worley et al., 2012
grsp-44 grsp-42 nlp-12 grsp-35 grsp-37 grsp-36 (5.13kb) grsp-43 fip-8 fip-6 fipr-26 (1.12kb) grsp-17 fipr-23 fipr-22 (2.19kb); grsp-33 grsp-29 (7.06kb) grsp-26 grsp-22 grsp-8 (4.91kb); nlp-32 grsp-9 cnc-6 (5.69kb) nlp-10 fipr-18 fip-3 fipr-16 fip-1(50.45kb) fipr-17 nlp-21 grsp-32(80.31kb); grsp-11 grsp-12 dct-8 (2.18kb) dct-7 grsp-13 grsp-14 grsp-21 (4.64kb) grsp-30 fipr-14 fipr-15 grsp-20 (12.39kb) grsp-41; grsp-23 cnc-11 cnc-1 cnc-5 cnc-4 cnc-3 cnc-2 (7.17kb) grsp-19 grsp-18 grsp-16 (8,41kb) nlp-34 nlp-31 nlp-30 nlp-29 nlp-28 nlp-27 (10.52kb) grsp-40 grsp-38 (1,05kb) grsp-45 grsp-10 cnc-9 grsp-31 fipr-11 fipr-10 fipr-12 (37,43kb) fipr-13 fipr-5 fipr-4 fipr-7 fipr-6 (10.23kb) nlp-33 cnc-10 (35.88kb) nlp-24 fipr-1 grsp-5 grsp-7 (42.73kb) grsp-27 grsp-6 nlp-25 nlp-26 (6,02kb) cnc-7; grsp-47 grsp-46 grsp-48 (3.16kb) fip-5 fipr-21 cnc-8 (3.88kb) grsp-15	*S.enterica*	Head & Aballay, 2014
grsp-42 nlp-12 grsp-35 grsp-37 grsp-36 (5.12kb) grsp-43 fipr-26 fipr-22 fipr-24 (2.16kb); grsp-33 grsp-29 grsp-28 (2.06kb) grsp-26 grsp-8; nlp-32 cnc-6 nlp-10 fip-1 fip-3 fipr-16 (48.96kb) fipr-17; fipr-30 dct-7 grsp-13 grsp-21(213.78kb) grsp-3 fipr-14 grsp-41; grsp-23 cnc-1 cnc-11 cnc-5 cnc-4 cnc-3 cnc-2 (5.75kb) grsp-19 grsp-16 (8.41kb) nlp-31 nlp-30 nlp-29 nlp-28 nlp-27 (9.24kb) fip-2 grsp-40 grsp-38 (1.05kb) grsp-45 grsp-4 grsp-31 fipr-4 fipr-5 fipr-6 fipr-7 fipr-8 fipr-9 (18.61kb) nlp-33 nlp-24 (469kb) grsp-5 grsp-7 (1.48kb) grsp-27 nlp-25 nlp-26 (6.02kb) cnc-7; grsp-47 grsp-46 grsp-48 (3.16kb) fip-5 fipr-21 cnc-8 (3.88kb)	*S. aureus*	Bond et al., 2014

Notes: Black letters: GRSPs were up-regulated. Blue letters: GRSPs were down-regulated. Co-expressed GRSP clusters were shadowed by grey. GRSPs on different chromosome were separated by a semicolon.

Table 3. Differential expression of GRSPs and co-expression of GRSPs clusters after *C. elegans* infection.

(for details, please refer to Table S4 in [12]). Certainly, it is possible that two *C. elegans* GRSPs (*grsp-24* and *grsp-39*) without detectable expression in previous studies analyzed here may be detectable in other studies, which we were unable to mine due to the limited length of this study [7].

3.6. The evolution of GRSPs multigene families by gene duplications

GRSPs subfamilies were classified based on the precursor sequences similarity and gene structure conservation. Phylogenetic analysis was performed using the signal peptide sequences. It is possible that the similarity between the two group sequences is not perfectly consistent among these GRSPs, which resulted in the observations that certain members within the same subfamilies were located in a different clade in the phylogenetic tree (**Figure 3**). Orthologous GRSPs of the two nematodes detected in the above could be well defined by phylogenetic analysis. Certain members of subfamilies (such as the members of subfamily I) were clustered together on their chromosomes and also the same clade on the phylogenetic tree (**Figure 3**). Five GRSPs from *nlp-27* to *nlp-31* were clustered on *C. elegans* genome. Phylogenetic analysis showed *nlp-27* clade was different from the clade formed by *nlp-28–nlp-31*, which was similar to previous results [7].

Subfamily	dN-dS	SE	Probability	R(Ti/Tv)
I	−5.323	0.073	0.000	1.81
II	−2.228	0.038	0.028	1.32
III	−3.626	0.087	0.011	1.21
IV	−3.321	0.035	0.000	5.54
V	−4.510	0.042	0.011	1.52
VI	−5.326	0.036	0.000	1.26
VII	−3.692	0.028	0.000	3.32
VIII	−2.649	0.053	0.022	1.78
IX	−3.451	0.038	0.000	1.67
X	−2.942	0.046	0.000	2.15
XI	−3.153	0.061	0.031	1.93
XII	−4.324	0.049	0.000	4.34
XIII	−3.256	0.027	0.000	1.52
XIV	−2.968	0.039	0.021	2.86

Notes: dN, non-synonymous substitutions; dS, synonymous substitutions; SE, standard error; Ti, transition; Tv, transversion; R, overall transition/transversion bias. The overall average difference of (dN-dS) was less than zero, and standard error value was less than 0.05.

Table 4. Estimates of overall average variance and pattern of nucleotide substitution.

3.7. Purifying selection of the two nematode GRSPs

Under the model of codon-based Z-test, the estimate of purifying selection was conducted directly to analyze sequence pairs and overall average. Its values are identically equal to zero and therefore rejected the null hypothesis of strict neutrality (dS = dN) and accepted the alternative hypothesis. The difference in average overall of dN-dS was less than zero. The standard error values were less than 0.05. Synonymous substitutions were clearly prevailing on protein-coding sequences of the nematode GRSPs, which indicated the occurrences of purifying selection. With an average ratio of R (Ti/Tv) > 1, the patterns of nucleotide substitution also showed a predominance of transitions over transversions (**Table 4**).

4. Discussion

Soil organisms (*A. thaliana*) and/or bacterial feeders (the two nematodes: *D. discoideum* and fruit fly, who feed on rotting fruit with a large number of bacteria) are relatively enriched for GRSPs in the current study. The environment and survival stress of soil living and/or bacterial feeding may be one of the main evolutionary driving forces for the expansion of lineage-specific GRSPs in the two nematodes. This was exemplified by the expansion of nematode-specific chemosensory genes (for *C. elegans* it is about 2000 and for human it is about 1000, about 2 times), which allowed it to mount a rapid response to environmental stimuli [17]. Comparing to the amplification of nematode-specific chemosensory genes, one may be more impressed by the amplification of nematode-specific GRSPs (for *C. elegans,* it is about 110 and for human, it is 4, about 28 times).

The conservation of precursor organizations, the unaltered position and phase of intron, together with the homologous sequence of DNA, suggested that the GRSPs clusters in the two nematodes might come from physically local DNA reproductions. The duplication of local genes came into being by gene clusters of paralogous genes whose products have similar functions. Paralogous genes with similar functions and expression patterns are frequent in *C. elegans* [18]. The co-expression of gene clusters encoding different proteins with similar functions in specific regions should provide effective combinatorial methods to coordinate complex biological systems [19]. The scales of most co-expression GRSPs clusters on their chromosomes are less than 10 kb and the smallest one is 1.05 kb (co-expression of *grsp-40* and *grsp-38*) (**Table 3**). Different GRSPs within the same cluster differentially responded to the same infection. For example, GRSPs from *cnc-1* to *cnc-5* (7.17 kb) and *cnc-11* in the same cluster showed co-expression with the upregulation of *cnc-11, cnc-1,* and *cnc-2* and the down-regulation from *cnc-3* to *cnc-5* after *C. elegans* infection [14]. GRSPs cluster from *grsp-35* to *grsp-36* (5.13 kb) were upregulated by *M. nematophilum* and *P. aeruginosa* infection of *C. elegans* [8, 16] and downregulated by *S. enterica* and *S. aureus* infection [13, 14]. A noticeable overlap of *C. elegans* GRSPs induced by different infections may indicate that the different sets of induced *C. elegans* GRSPs may still share some functionalities. Considering a large amount of operon regulation in *C. elegans,* we analyzed all *C. elegans* genes contained within operon by an internal Perl Scripts search to detect whether the small clusters of adjacent GRSPs could be co-regulated by operon regulation. While no *C. elegans* GRSPs were identified in operon regions (data not shown), the short genetic and physical distance on chromosomes and highly homologous sequences suggest that neighboring GRSPs arising from duplicated GRSPs may share the same regulatory sequences. The same regulatory sequences on their promoters can be directly and coordinately activated by transcription factors binding to the shared regulatory elements.

With similar variance of (dn-dS), the two nematode GRSPs might have experienced similar selective stress during evolution, which is in concordance with the neutral mutation-random drift theory of molecular evolution. Relative conserved synteny blocks of the GRSPs orthologous clusters suggested that these GRSPs were subjected to functional restraint. With the increasing species complexity, the genome size and the members of a gene family usually undergo an evolutionary expansion in abundance for similar essential basic cellular mechanisms shared by eukaryotes [20]. The basic physiological process for *C. elegans* is similar to those observed in higher organisms. Few matching orthologs of *C. elegans* GRSPs in the other species may indirectly reflect nematode-specific biological functions of *C. elegans* GRSPs that are essential for nematode-specific environments such as soil living and bacterial feeding. The evolutionary diversification of these GRSPs might enhance the ability of *C. elegans* innate immunity to adapt to environmental stress [7].

This study built a full set of GRSPs from the algae *G. theta* to the mammal human by genome-wide comparison across 10 species. The two nematodes were enriched for GRSPs, which demonstrated a good example of DNA local reproductions and maintained a relative conserved synteny block on their genomes after speciation and separation. The phylogenetic conservation of synteny GRSPs clusters on their genomes, the co-expressed GRSPs clusters, and strong purifying selection may indicate evolutionary constraints acting on *C. elegans* to guarantee that *C. elegans* could mount a rapid systematical response to infection by co-expression of GRSPs clusters on the genomes. The mechanism of co-expression, co-regulation, and co-functionality behind these GRSPs clusters is still unknown. Our knowledge about it is expected to improve by the increasing comparative genomics of correlated expression patterns across different nematodes (such as *C. brenneri* and *C. remanei*), which holds promise to provide insights into the adaptive advantage of co-expressed GRSPs in nematodes.

Acknowledgements

This work was supported by grants from the National Nature Science Foundation of China (31160233), the Science and Technology Foundation of Jiangxi Province (20142BAB204013).

Author details

Muying Ying*, Mingyue Ren, Chenglin Liu and Ping Zhao

*Address all correspondence to: yingmuying@ncu.edu.cn

Department of Molecular Biology and Biochemistry, Basic Medical College of Nanchang University, Nanchang, PR China

References

[1] Tang SJ, Sun KH, Sun GH, Lin G, Lin WW, Chuang MJ. Cold-induced ependymin expression in zebrafish and carp brain: implications for cold acclimation. FEBS Letters. 1999;**459**:95-99. DOI: 10.1016/S0014-5793(99)01229-6

[2] Khan I, Maldonado E, Vasconcelos V, O&Brien SJ, Johnson WE, Antunes A. Mammalian keratin associated proteins (KRTAPs) subgenomes: Disentangling hair diversity and adaptation to terrestrial and aquatic environments. BMC Genomics. 2014;**15**:779. DOI: 10.1186/1471-2164-15-779

[3] Ciuzan O, Hancock J, Pamfil D, Wilson I, Ladomery M. The evolutionarily conserved multifunctional glycine-rich RNA binding proteins play key roles in development and stress adaptation. Physiologia Plantarum. 2015;**153**:1-11. doi: 10.1111/ppl.12286

[4] Mangeon A, Jungueira RM, Sachetto-Martins G. Functional diversity of the plant glycine-rich proteins superfamily. Plant Signaling & Behaviour. 2010;**5**:99-104

[5] Mallo GV, Kurz C, Couillault C, Pujol N, Granjeaud S, Kohara Y, Ewbank JJ. Inducible antibacterial defense system in *C. elegans*. Current Biology. 2002;**12**:1209-1214. DOI: 10.1016/S0960-9822(02)00928-4

[6] Couillault C, Pujol N, Reboul J, Sabatier L, Guichou JF, Kohara Y, Ewbank JJ. TLR-independent control of innate immunity in *Caenorhabditis elegans* by the TIR domain adaptor protein TIR-1, an ortholog of human SARM. Nature Immunology. 2004;**5**:488-494. DOI: 10.1038/ni1060

[7] Pujol N, Zugasti O, Wong D, Couillault C, Kurz CL, Schulenburg H, Ewbank JJ. Antifungal innate immunity in *C. elegans* is enhanced by evolutionary diversification of antimicrobial peptides. PLoS Pathogens. 2008;**4**:e1000105. DOI: 10.1371/journal.ppat.1000105

[8] O&Rourke D, Baban D, Demidova M, Mott R, Hodgkin J. Genomic clusters, putative pathogen recognition molecules, and antimicrobial genes are induced by infection of *C. elegans* with *M. nematophilum*. Genome Research. 2006;**16**:1005-1016. DOI: 10.1101/gr.50823006

[9] Krzywinski M, Schein J, Birol I, Connors J, Gascoyne R, Horsman D, Jones SJ, Marra MA. Circos: An information aesthetic for comparative genomics. Genome Research. 2009;**19**:1639-1645. doi: 10.1101/gr.092759.109

[10] Tamura K, Stecher G, Peterson D, Filipski A, Kumar S. MEGA6: Molecular evolutionary genetics analysis version 6.0. Molecular Biology and Evolution. 2013;**30**:2725-2729. DOI: 10.1093/molbev/mst197

[11] Pearson WR, Robins G, Zhang T. Generalized neighbor-joining: More reliable phylogenetic tree reconstruction. Molecular Biology and Evolution. 1999;**16**:806-816. DOI: 10.1007/978-1-62703-646-7_5

[12] Ying M, Qiao Y, Yu L. Evolutionary expansion of nematode-specific glycine-rich secreted peptides. Gene. 2016;**587**:76-82. DOI: 10.1016/j.gene.2016.04.049

[13] Bond MR, Ghosh S, Wang P, Hanover JA. Conserved nutrient sensor O-GlcNAc transferase is integral to *C. elegans* pathogen-specific immunity. PLoS One. 2014;**9**:e113231. DOI: 10.1371/journal.pone.0113231

[14] Head B, Aballay A. Recovery from an acute infection in *C. elegans* requires the GATA transcription factor ELT-2. PLoS Genetics. 2014;**10**:e1004609. DOI: 10.1371/journal.pgen.1004609

[15] Pukkila-Worley R, Rhonda FR, Kirienko NV, Larkins-Ford J, Conery AL, Ausubel FM. Stimulation of host immune defenses by a small molecule protects *C. elegans* from bacterial infection. PLoS Genetics. 2012;**8**:e1002733. DOI: 10.1371/journal.pgen.1002733

[16] Sun J, Singh V, Kajino-Sakamoto R, Aballay A. Neuronal GPCR controls innate immunity by regulating noncanonical unfolded protein response genes. Science. 2011;**332**:729-732. DOI: 10.1126/science.1203411

[17] Bargmann CI. Chemosensation in *C. elegans*. WormBook. 2006;**25**:1-29. DOI: 10.1895/wormbook.1.123.1

[18] *C. elegans* Sequencing Consortium. Genome sequence of the nematode *C. elegans*: a platform for investigating biology. Science. 1998;**282**:2012-2018. DOI: 10.1126/science.282.5396.2012

[19] Sugimoto A. High-throughput RNAi in *Caenorhabditis elegans*: genome-wide screens and functional genomics. Differentiation. 2004;**72**:81-91. DOI: 10.1111/j.1432-0436.2004.07202004.x

[20] Ying M, Huang X, Zhao H, Wu Y, Wan F, Huang C, Jie K. Comprehensively surveying structure and function of RING domains from *Drosophila melanogaster*. PLoS One. 2011;**6**:e23863. DOI: 10.1371/journal.pone.0023863

Chapter 6

Assessing the Viability and Degeneration of the Medically Important Filarial Nematodes

Charles D. Mackenzie, Ashley Behan-Braman,
Joe Hauptman and Timothy Geary

Additional information is available at the end of the chapter

http://dx.doi.org/10.5772/intechopen.69512

Abstract

The assessment of nematodes as they generate and die is not a simple thing to do due in part to the complexity of the organism, and the fact that still relatively little is known about their physiology and internal biology. Indeed, the pathological changes in the internal organs of the worms are still only recognized in general terms. Obviously dead worms are easily recognized (when fractured, or calcified, etc.) but the lesser obvious changes can be difficult to detect and interpret. The point at which a worm can be defined as dead is not a simple matter; cessation of motility is currently the most commonly used parameter for this but it is not always a robust indicator and better indicators are needed. Various methods can be used to assess the presence, viability, and functionality of nematodes but these must be used with an understanding of the situation at hand and the specific questions being addressed. Careful use of appropriate statistics is essential given the complex nature of the target organism and the variability in the changes that can be seen within even one anatomical component of these worms. Histological assessment of the parasites present in both parasitized host tissues and isolated worms used in *in vitro* experiments can provide information that gives a more detailed understanding of the changes in nematodes as they degenerate and die. Understanding of the pathways nematodes follows as they degenerate naturally or under various external pressures, such as chemotherapy, remains a fascinating and potentially productive goal for investigation. Likewise, a complete understanding and definition of specific indicators that reflect parasite load, parasite viability, and damage, or reduced fecundity, will greatly help the fight against those nematode infections that currently cause significant burdens of disease in humans and animals.

Keywords: filarial nematodes, assessment, viability, death, histopathology

INTECH
open science | open minds

1. Introduction

Nematodes commonly infect humans, animals, and plants in all the ecosystems from the tropics to the polar regions; they can cause significant damage and consequently are responsible for some of the major chronic infections of these hosts. This being the case there is a great need to develop better treatment and prophylactic procedures to reduce the pathological effects of these infections, much of which are caused by events associated with the degeneration and death of the causative parasites in sensitive host tissues. Successful development of new effective and safe chemotherapeutic agents, a leading approach in controlling these detrimental effects, necessarily requires improved and more accurate assessment of the viability of these organisms. This is needed to both develop control mechanisms as well as to determine the epidemiological nature of these parasites.

In general terms, much is known about the effects of many parasitic nematodes on their human and animal hosts but comparatively little about the effects of the hosts, or chemotherapeutic agents, on the parasites themselves, i.e. the pathology of the parasites. There is, however increasing knowledge about model nematodes such as *Caenorhabditis elegans*, but still in comparison very little is known about the detailed biology and pathobiology of the more complex nematodes that commonly infect humans, animals, and plants; nor is it clear how useful it is to compare the model nematode, *C. elegans,* with the parasitic nematodes. A better understanding of these parasites in terms of their vital functions and their various pathophysiological changes - such as their mode of nutrition, the internal changes that lead irreversibly to their death, and the definition of specific parameters that indicate their viability - are essential to progress in this important field of research and development. Improved methods of controlling parasitic nematodes have the potential of improving the medical care of millions of humans and animals, as well greatly improving the yields of production crops.

Many examples exist in disease management suggest that it is important that we gain a clearer understanding of the biology of the infecting nematodes and the effects that the host and drugs induce in these parasites. Plant parasitic nematodes cause very significant problems to major crops throughout the world including vegetables, fruits and grain crops [1]. Some of the most devastating of chronic tropical diseases in human medicine are caused by nematodes; indeed, a major global health effort has been underway for some years aimed to control and eliminating a few of these tropical diseases. Two of the most successful programs today involve filarial nematodes, one that causes "river blindness" (onchocerciasis) and a second that is responsible for "tropical elephantiasis" (lymphatic filariasis). Well over 100 million people are affected by these parasites, and many more people still are at risk of these infections. The veterinary world has long understood the importance of parasitic infections, especially the persistent intestinal nematode parasites, with their ability to compromise growth and development of domestic animals. In both human and animal infections, the primary approach to reduce and eliminate these parasites has been for almost a century using chemotherapeutic agents - agents that either primarily damage and destroy the infecting organism, an event that can often induce a reactive pathological response in the host, especially with tissue based nematodes.

Central to measuring, understanding and treating parasitic infections in animals and humans are two fundamental parameters–worm load (i.e. number) and the worm viability; for many years, these have been assessed by active counting the number of viable worms (or a more easily detectable parasitic stage such as eggs, etc.) present in the host. Nematode infections in humans and animals that cause significant disease are essentially found in three major locations: in organs (e.g. digestive and respiratory tract lumens and ducts), in connective tissues, or in the circulatory vessels (lymphatics and blood vessels). Those parasites that lie in the gut are perhaps the most well-known and in many ways the most studied in human and animals, and are arguably more commonly seen because their cycles include detectable faecal stages. Thus, the time-honored test for assessing loads of these parasites has been the measurement of their egg production by the parasites (i.e. fecal egg counts through a variety of well-described methods: McMaster, Kato-Katz, mini-Flotac and other various egg concentrating methods) [2–5]. In recent years, there has been the gradual development and validation of molecular (PCR) approaches for estimating intestinal nematode presence and load, and it is likely that this type of technique will be used more commonly in the future.

In the case of *in vitro* experiments direct observations, such as motility, are used to distinguish between live and dead worms. This latter procedure, which appears at first glance to be relatively easy, is in fact not necessarily so, and thus there is a need to better understand the processes and indicators that are associated with the degeneration and death of parasitic nematodes. In more recent years other indicators of infection such as the presence of specific antibodies and circulating antigens derived from the worms have entered into the diagnostic menu; currently, an even wider range of indirect indicators of infection, such as parasite-derived microRNAs, are being investigated. In this present chapter, we will focus more specifically the issue of defining the viability of parasitic nematodes through direct means rather than the wider area of clinical diagnosis. We use as our model filarial nematodes which, are as described above important human and animal parasites, and where the major intervention used to control and eliminate these infections in medical terms is chemotherapy.

2. Filarial nematodes

Filariae are a very diverse group of nematodes that infect a very wide range of specific hosts. The three major filarial human nematode infections are river blindness or onchocerciasis (*Onchocerca volvulus*), lymphatic filariasis (*Wuchereria bancrofti* and *Brugia* sp.) and loiasis (*Loa loa*). In canines, *Dirofilaria sp.* are the most important filarial nematodes, and exists in most areas of the world. The filarial nematodes we will refer to in our discussion here focused on a morphological approach to assessing nematode viability are found naturally either in the major lymphatics and blood vessels (*Brugia* sp.), or in tissues and small vessels of connective tissues (*Onchocerca* sp.). The transmission these filarial parasites involves blood-sucking vectors, and the life spans comparatively long for the adult worms (5–12 years); their life cycles are depicted in summary in **Figure 1**.

Filarial worms are one of the best examples of a group of parasitic nematodes where a better understanding of the biological status of the parasite, or at least of certain parasitic stages, is

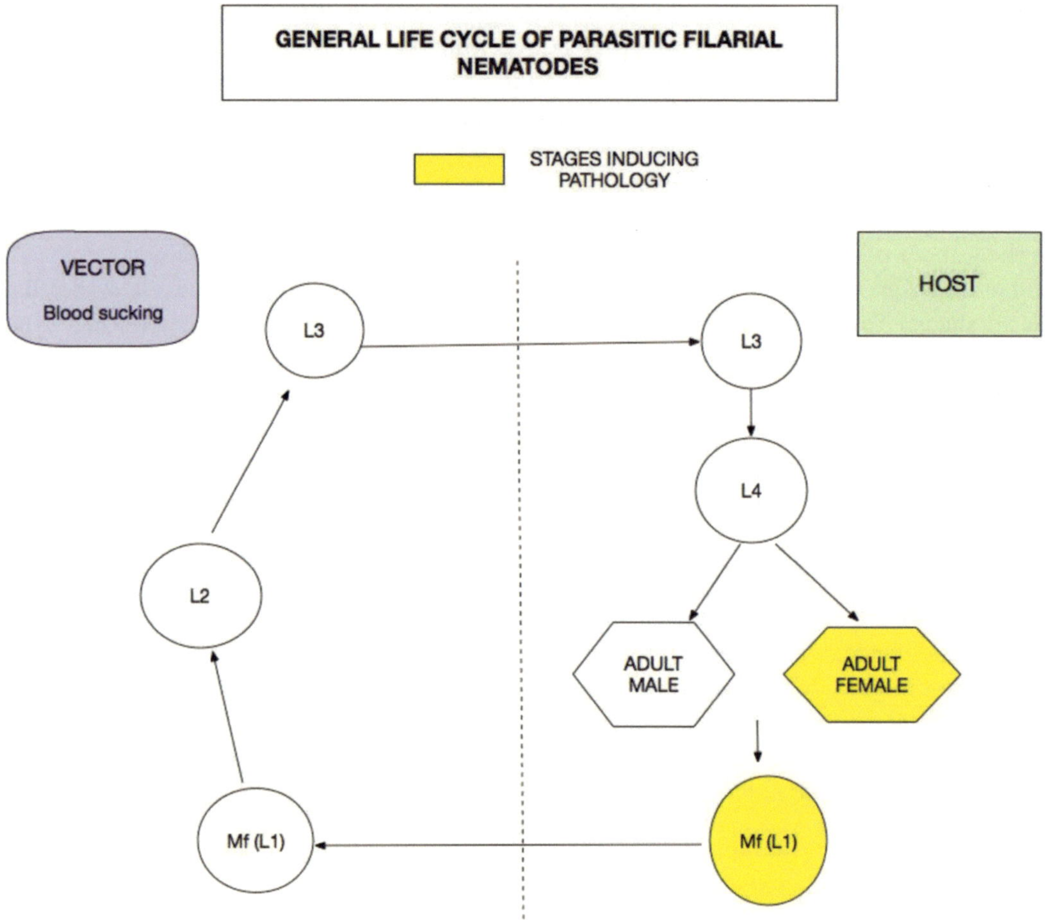

Figure 1. The general life cycle of parasitic filarial worms.

essential to establishing optimal effective and safe therapies, and to obtain a clearer understanding the pathogenesis of the disease in the host. Such an increased understanding is particularly important since these parasites infect and effect internal tissues such as connective tissues and circulatory vessels; this makes them more difficult targets for control compared to those nematodes that reside in the intestine where often treatment results in complete rejection of the damaged organism from the body.

3. Assessment of parasitic nematodes

In assessing a nematode infection in a host, it is important to select the most appropriate stage of these five-stage parasites to focus on and use as an indicator. This depends very much on the life-cycle in the host, as well as the availability of suitable techniques for assessment. For example, if one is trying to break infection transmission to a vector then the crucial stage that provides the most important information in terms of epidemiological control is usually the stage entering the vector; in the filarial infections, this is almost exclusively the microfilarial stage. However, it is possible that permanent alterations in an earlier phase or stage may also be a strong and useful indicator that can predict termination of transmission. In our example here, evidence of a destroyed capability to reproduce and produce the first stage forms (the microfilariae) seen in significant uterine damage, and thus a lack of production of microfilariae, is an important indicator of the breaking of transmission. Observing such changes in adult female worms may indeed be more practically feasible than detecting the presence of transmissible microfilariae in the host or in the blood-feeding vectors. The effective break in the parasite's cycle, seen here in the permanent uterine damage and ceased reproductive ability, also shows that the actual death of the female worm is not the necessary target endpoint for defining a successful therapeutic agent or intervention: female worms may still be thought to be alive but have permanently lost the capability of reproducing. This also demonstrates the fact the simple counting of worm numbers often needs to be supported by an assessment of the internal anatomy of worms (e.g. the uteri or other vital structures) rather than just the number of whole worms present; a sterile worm is functionally as important as a dead worm. Thus, it is important to have methods of assessing the functional anatomy of worms. In both gut-residing nematodes and the tissue/vessel filariae, it is arguably more important to understand the functional state and reproductive capability of adult worms than just their physical, or numerical, presence. Measuring such parameters can either be done through histopathology examination as described below, or by the identification of products from components of the worms such as the uterus that may be released and be able to be detected in body fluids.

Assessment of the reproductive organs of male worms may also be a useful target for assessment; male filarial parasites are in the minority, and are probably fertilizing more than one female. Given that the reproductive cycle of filariae is comparatively long (months), it is likely that the female–the producer of the transmissible stage–is overall a better indicator of the host's infection status than is the male. The other stages that occur in hosts after infection, the third and fourth parasitic stages, are in general both hard to detect physically and exist for relatively short periods compared to the other stages; they have not been to date very useful targets for parasitological assessment. However, an indirect assessment of these stages through stage-specific antibodies or specific circulating antigens is becoming more feasible as the reagents for this type of test are improving rapidly.

It is important to re-emphasize, in the context of monitoring nematode infections, the distinction between using functional parameters and assessment that is through simple numerical quantification. In most cases a more detailed assessment that involves more functional parameters (biochemistry, fecundity etc.) is preferable. However, an exception where an estimation of the circulating load of the parasite is crucial and preferred is loiasis, caused by the filarial nematode *Loa loa*. This is a disease that appears to cause relatively little pathology except following the administration of ivermectin or diethylcarbamazine, anti-filarial drugs that are commonly used in treating filariasis. When these drugs are administered to individuals who carry high loads of circulating microfilariae their blood (>20,000 microfilariae/ml) severe reactions can occur and there is an increase of these people dying or being permanently affected due to vascular damage in their CNS tissues. It is, therefore, crucial that before treating with the two drugs mentioned above the number of circulating parasites (the parasitic load) in their blood must be known. It is, in this case, not a matter of whether these parasites are functional (e.g. are able to be taken up by the vector and continue the life cycle), but what is the load of worms present and this done often by a standard blood smear estimation. The newly developed systems for measuring worm loads in blood improves the reproducibility and practicality when sampling in comparatively difficult situations such as in the field. Systems based on iPhone imaging technology (the LoaScope), and other utilizing light-scattering principles (the WiggleTron) [6], can now rapidly measure the number of parasites in blood smears at the field laboratory level.

The most common approach to assessing the viability of worms *in vitro* is through direct observation of their motion, commonly by visual means although image analysis systems have been developed. Motility has been used in numerous studies and has been the major approach used for the assessment chemotherapeutic agents for over 40 years. There are however the number of drawbacks at play using this approach including observer to observer variation, the lack of consistency of parasites' movement–often nematodes, including filariae, can be unable to move due to various local environmental reasons, such as inadequate culture fluid quality and sub-optimal temperature. However, arguably the most important challenge with using this technique is a lack of definition concerning the relationship between immotility and actual death of the worm. Techniques have been developed to improve the observation of motility in nematodes. For example, as the motion of most healthy nematodes follows a common repeatable pattern it is possible to detect alterations in these using detection systems that take many estimations of motion pattern over a short period of time. The "Wiggletron" system is one of these, a technique based on the recording of light deflected by the worms' motion, has improved the consistency of measuring worm motility *in vitro* and has been used to document the effects of various chemotherapeutic agents on filariae [6].

Deciding on the optimal means of assessing worm viability and number requires a consideration of the specific question being addressed, as well as the circumstances at hand. As mentioned above assessing nematodes *in vivo*, such as those present in tissues in or from infected individuals, usually requires a somewhat different approach from that need to investigate nematodes *in vitro*. A major challenge that must be addressed with studying this organism *in vitro* is that no robust culture system has been developed yet for filariae. Parasites used *in vitro* have inevitably come from an *in vivo* origin and may have already been affected by their status in their originating host, and are then placed in a compromised environment even before the test conditions are applied; this fact is often problematic in studies that look for degeneration and pathological changes in the worms. Understanding the genesis and form of subtle anatomic changes in such worms is therefore very important. Another complicating factor with filariae, both for *in vitro* or *in vivo* studies, is the fact that these worms are comparatively large and long. It is known that distinct degenerative changes can be in only one or two small sections of these long organisms and other areas in the same organ be quite normal, and thus it is relatively easy to fall foul of sampling error. Samples that statistically include a range of areas or sections in the worm are necessary for histological studies and the like. Similarly, motility–perhaps the currently most used parameter of "health" *in vitro* and indeed often used as a surrogate for the death of the nematodes–can be misleading with worms lying motionless to visual observation for long periods of time and then be seen to move again. More sensitive techniques that reveal, in a statistically robust manner, the type of motion that worms show over a longer time-period for example, do address this challenge to some extent. It is perhaps obvious to underscore here that in investigations of effects on filarial worms the parallel use of control samples is always essential, especially with *in vitro* experiments where the culture systems are less than perfect.

4. Technical aspects of assessing nematodes

The various techniques used to assess nematodes infections *in vivo* and worms that are maintained in vitro are summarized in **Figure 2**. The methods discussed here are focused on filarial worms, mainly because this is a parasite that has been the center of much of the recent research into better methods of controlling infections in humans. This is not to imply that there has also been a body of solid work in the same vein carried out in other disciplines, such as in plant pathology. The discussion here is focused on directly assessing worms themselves rather than the more indirect approaches through "footprint" surrogates such as antibody responses and circulating antigen.

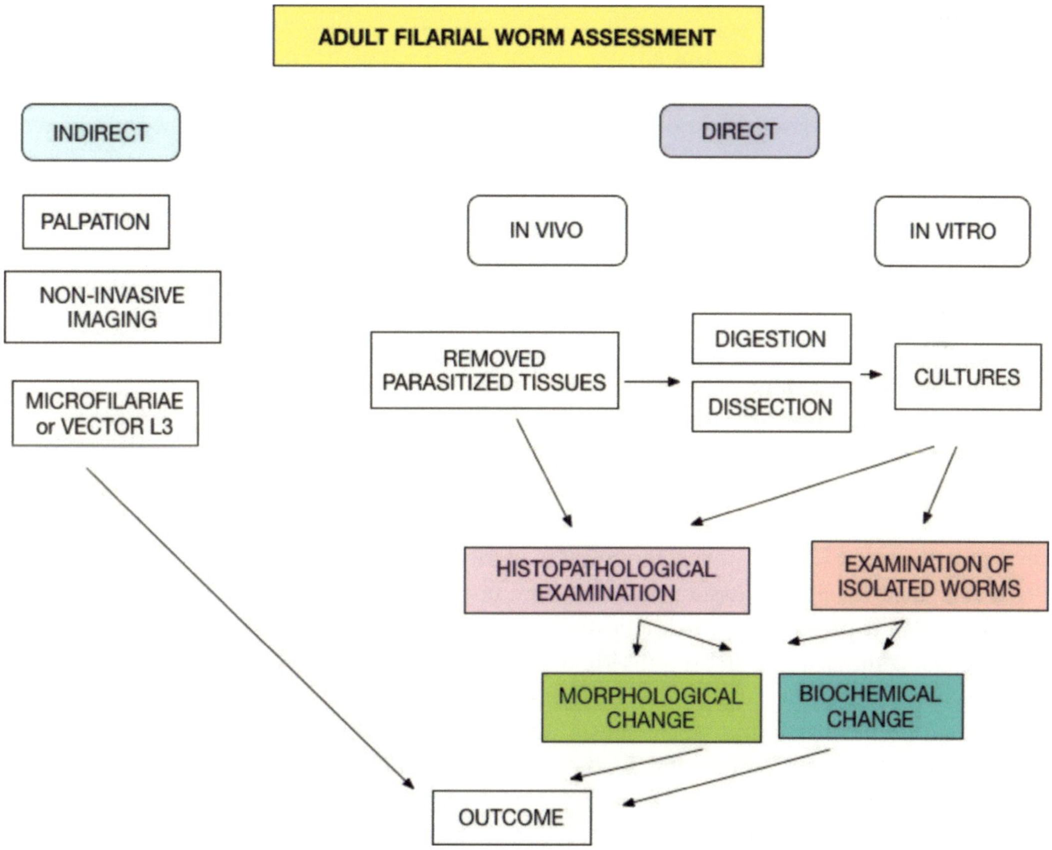

Figure 2. Assessing the status of filarial infections and filarial worms.

4.1. Indirect (clinical) assessment of population endemicity

Adult worms are central to the assessment the longevity of nematode infections, and this is particularly so in filarial infections, e.g. over five years with most filariae. The female adult worm is often used as the indicator worm rather than males because of its potential to produce large numbers of offspring and its remarkable longevity–arguably over 12 years in the case of *O. volvulus*. In assessing adult filarial worms *in vivo* there are several challenges. Although there is a site of anatomical predilection, in the case of LF it is the inguinal and femoral lymphatics, this is certainly not the only place these adult worms are found in the body. In onchocerciasis, the adults are found in "nodules" most commonly located in the pelvic girdle area (especially the iliac crest), but again can be found elsewhere such as on the chest wall and on the skull (the latter being more common in the children). *Onchocerca* nodules essentially are a nest of worms surrounded by fibrous inflammatory tissue. There have been very few autopsies carried out on individuals infected with this parasite but in the few that have been done these parasitized fibrous nodules have been found in the deep tissues along the femur bone, even when no externally palpable nodules are detected in the skin. Thus, although the presence of palpable nodules is arguably a good indicator at an epidemiological level it is not a particularly reliable indicator of individual infections. Currently, either the presence of microfilariae in the skin or eye, or a positive test to parasite-specific antibody remains the diagnostic tools of choice. With loiasis the adult worms can essentially be present anywhere on the body lying in the subcutaneous tissues and are known to migrate frequently under the skin, and in the external eye; in fact, loiasis is characteristically known for the fact that the adult worms can sometimes be seen migrating across the conjunctiva of the eye, hence the name "eye worm".

Therefore, manual palpation and clinical examination by experienced observers can be used to detect certain specific presentations of the main two filarial infections under discussion, with at least a moderate degree of reliability. The most reliable test being the assessment of the typical subcutaneous "nodules" (containing coiled adult worms and host inflammatory cells and tissues) in onchocerciasis; their presence in people living in a known endemic area has been to estimate the level of endemicity in the population of a defined geographic area. There are other causes of dermal nodules (e.g. dermal cysts, cysticercosis), but the typical location of onchocercal nodules on the body (iliac crest, the base of the spine, the chest wall or the head) increases the likelihood that such a mass is due to *O. volvulus.* The presence of nodules in adults has been used as an epidemiological indicator to catalyze the start of new chemotherapy control programs in endemic countries. Although it is highly likely that adult worms of this infection are also present in deeper tissues and therefore not able to be palpated, it is still likely that assessment of the prevalence of palpable nodules does reflect an acceptable degree a load of this parasite in a community or in an individual. In lymphatic filariasis swellings or lumps due to the presence of the adult parasite can be detected in the spermatic cord of infected males; these lumps (or 'nodules') are adult worm "nests": like onchocerciasis, these involve fibrous chronic inflammatory responses around the dead adult worms. These indirect reflections of infection are subject to misdiagnosis and are therefore often of limited diagnostic potential. However, their presence can greatly assist in interpreting any more general clinical signs of diseases that might be present in an individual; thus, the presence of typical nodules improves the diagnosis of onchocerciasis and lymphatic filariasis and the initiation of treatment.

http://dx.doi.org/10.5772/intechopen.69512

4.2. Imaging of parasites *in vivo*

There are certain specific occasions in filarial infections where the adult worms can be seen by careful direct observation or using a diagnostic instrument. Loiasis has often been identified in people through the observation by the patient themselves of the migrating adult worm passing across the conjunctiva of the eye (thereby giving this parasite the common name "eye worm"). Questionnaire-based surveys using photographs of these worms active in the eye have been used with endemic populations to estimate the degree of endemicity of geographic area; such a frightening experience as watching a several centimeters long parasite pass across one's external eye–for example with women using a mirror to put on makeup in the morning–is dramatically memorable. Another example of the use of direct observation of the presence of worms is the identification by ophthalmologists using Slit Lamps to detect and count *Onchocerca* microfilariae present in the anterior chamber fluid of the human eye; in heavy infections almost 100 parasites can be present in this location–the observing of a 'Medusa's head" coiled mass of actively moving parasites in this location is not only dramatic and memorable but also provides a direct indication of the viability of the infecting parasites. Similarly using this ophthalmological instrument, or the simpler ophthalmoscopy, these microfilariae can also be seen lying within the cornea of the eye, often in association with small, usually whitish host reactions known as punctate keratitic spots; this is an example of where the death and degeneration of microfilariae can be directly observed and recorded.

Another non-invasive technique that has been used in both onchocerciasis and lymphatic filariasis to observe the movement of worms, and thus their presence and viability, is ultrasound imaging. Motile adult worms can be visualized in the lymphatic vessels of the inguinal canal of males infected with *W. bancrofti*, and likewise motile adult worms can be seen in the subcutaneous *O. volvulus* nodules–although the latter is less easy due to the worms here lying in tightly bound connective tissue rather than the intravascular location of the LF worms. Nevertheless, ultrasound is a technique that can assist both diagnosis and interpretation of the effects of chemotherapeutic interventions; however, it should be noted that this technique is relatively insensitive and best used as a supporting approach rather than the sole indicator in comparative studies. Recently developed techniques such OCT (optical coherence tomography) may be more sensitive.

4.3. Histopathological examination of infected host tissues

The histological assessment of parasite-containing tissues removed from patients is a very commonly used approach for assessing tissue (i.e. internally located) parasites, the subcutaneous nodules in onchocerciasis being a prime example in this present discussion. Most well-trained pathologists can identify the presence of a parasite in these tissues and do this by using some very simple characteristics that indicate the infecting organism (such as obvious outer walls containing non-mammalian cells), or by typical signs of a specific host reaction to these nematodes i.e. eosinophil and macrophage dominant host inflammatory responses. The viability status of the infecting nematode is usually only classified through major changes (e.g. its overall anatomical integrity, the breaking of the parasite wall, calcification etc.). More subtle changes in the parasite as it degenerates are still much less understood, therefore much less described in regular histopathological reports of parasite-induced pathology. Nevertheless, such histopathological material is a vital window that can be used to describe the biology of the worm and its own pathology as it degenerates and dies. A good example is seen in advances in the understanding of the biology of many nematodes that has come in recent years from histological studies of the filarial endosymbiont *Wolbachia.* However, relatively little is described about other aspects of the changing anatomy in filarial worms as they degenerate, die and undergo pathological changes; nor is there much described with any of the parasitic nematodes. The careful examination of morphological changes within worms, either those *in situ* taken from infected hosts or those that have been exposed to drugs *in vitro,* is needed to develop a better understanding of the viability and state of degeneration of the worm, and will lead to more informative research findings, certainly more robust results than are produced from the simple recording of motility.

One of the characteristics of filarial nematodes that has inhibited studies at the histological level is the fact that these organisms are comparatively long and very narrow; the name "filarial" comes from the Latin word for "thread". There are many anatomical differences at different places along this almost 200–300 μm long adult worm. Indeed, it has been noted that the degree of change and degeneration in these worms can vary considerably from place to place within a single worm; this makes an assessment of developing degenerative changes in the worms hard to detect unless the worm has reached the stage of almost complete anatomical degeneration and the whole organism is changed. The more subtle changes that take place within this long organism as it progresses and degenerates towards obvious physical finality are poorly described to date. In fact, what change or changes that can be defined as the irreversible point(s) of degeneration of the worm remains unclear, and indeed may vary from species to species.

Many of the early morphological studies on the effects of drugs on filariae were focused on electron microscopic (EM) studies and although changes were seen using this technique, observations such as these (which are carried out at a very high power magnification) are notoriously poor for defining the overall changes in the observed worm or a group of worms. EM images usually only look at a very small proportion of the worm's complex anatomy, and thus do not give a good overall assessment of the status of the whole organism. Such detailed level techniques are however useful for defining specific anatomical characteristics such as those of the endosymbiont bacteria *Wolbachia pipiens;* electron microscopic studies and several immunochemical descriptions of these important organisms do exist in the literature.

A characteristic that has often being sought in filarial worms, and particularly with worms in adult filarial worm nests, is the age of the worm or worms being observed; such information with these long living worms is useful to those studying epidemiological questions. As these parasites ingest blood, and the products of its breakdown accumulate in the parasite's intestines over time, the presence of hemosiderin (often defined histochemically) in the gut has been used as an indicator of an older worm. Degeneration has been commonly defined by simple anatomical change although some histological markers, usually immunomarkers, have been used to reflect biochemical degeneration. One such example is the reduction in the molecule Nras, an important component in cell cycle maintenance, which occurs in adult female *O. volvulus* worms under the long-term pressure of *in vivo* chemotherapy with the anthelminthic ivermectin [7].

There is a major challenge in making statistically relevant observations on nematodes, organisms that have a lengthy anatomy and that often are coiled *in vivo*. Histopathological sections of onchocercal nodules naturally pass through several individual worms present in such coils and the identification of individual worms is not reliably feasible in most cases. It is statistically much more appropriate to regard each nest of worms as a single statistical entity, and assess the status of a whole nodule by observing and scoring the histological section as a whole; and in fact, to assess at least three 2–3 mm separated sections in a standard nodule of approximately 1 cm diameter; more slices may be needed depending on the parameter being assayed and the statistical power of the study in question. Various basic histochemical stains have been used with histological sections of parasite and the essentially routine stains, such as hematoxylin and eosin, together with stains that identifying certain chemical components such as carbohydrates, usually can provide substantial amounts of morphological evidence of change.

A caution must also be made here in that although nodules are usually removed by the surgeons as "single usually ovoid" structures, or collection of ovoid structures in heavy infections, and then these masses typically bisected through the longest axis for histopathological and other studies. These "halves" are not always equivalent in parasitic content; it has been noted that after long-term use of ivermectin the remaining adult worms often clustered in nests to one side of the ovoid nodule rather than being in the center as seen in untreated nodules. Thus, simple bisection does not necessarily provide equal content in these cases, and if one is bisecting a nodule to use two different assays to determining worm status–for example one-half for pathology and the other for molecular assay,–one cannot assume that the two halves are equal of similar in terms of parasitic content.

These basic principles in the preparation and assessment of onchocercal nodules (**Figure 3**) also apply to the examination of worm nests in lymphatic filariasis, although this is rarely done in human infections it is used in experimental models and in studies of other natural filarial infections where the worms are present in nests and nodules a such a *Onchocerca* sp. (e.g. *Onchocerca ochengi*) in cattle.

4.4. Isolation of worms from host tissues

In the case of onchocerciasis, the surgical removal of the fibrous subcutaneous nodules, and is in fact regarded as a therapeutic step, as it removes at least some of the fecund females; removal of nodules is also in some cases also a definitive diagnostic step. In many field situations, material collected this way also provides the opportunity for assessment of the viability of the worms in these nodules. This approach remains one of few readily available approaches to assessing the presence and status of worms *in vivo,* and for many studies it has also provided isolated adult worms for additional *in vitro* studies–the worms for these investigations being isolated either by careful manual dissection or by digestion of the fibrous host tissues using enzymes.

As these parasites are embedded in chronic host inflammatory responses, which in the case of filarial parasites usually contains a large amount of collagen, the general approach utilized for isolation is the use of enzymes to digest the worms free from the tissue. The most commonly

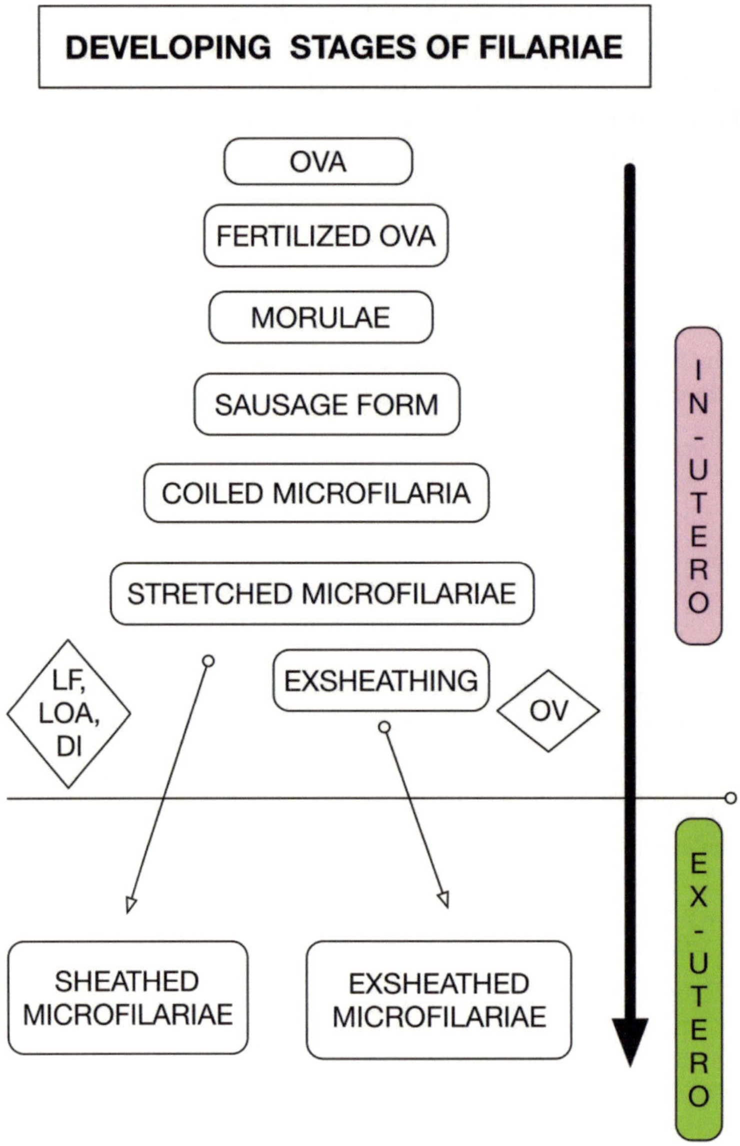

Figure 3. Methodology for preparing parasitized tissues and filarial worms for histological examination.

used enzyme is collagenase which targets the fibrous material [8]; the addition of dispase, a protease which targets fibronectin, collagen IV, and to a lesser extent collagen, is beneficial. It usually takes some 10–12 h to free the parasites in the case of *O. volvulus* nodules. This digestive process nevertheless can, and usually does, compromise many of the components of the worm themselves, although the major components such as the early uterine stages of microfilariae can be isolated from the digestates and easily counted. The re-implantation of cultured worms has also been used as an additional approach to testing viability [9, 10].

4.5. Assessing the changes in parasites

Alterations in worms that are extensively changed can often be seen by directly looking at the whole worm either *in situ* or *in vivo*. A typical sign of degeneration includes obvious breakage or decreased transparency (usually due to the degeneration of internal components and the accumulation of pathological constituents, e.g. calcification). In cases where there is severe damage with breakage or a marked increase density of the worms, it is likely that these worms are irreversibly damaged and this assessment requires only a simple examination with the naked eye. However, in some cases this visible degeneration is confined to only certain segments of the worm whereas other areas appear still viable and visually normal; care is therefore always needed in defining damage and the observing of the whole worm is essential (**Figure 4**).

It is the more subtle changes in nematodes that need better description and understanding of their significance. It is essential in this goal to understand the normal anatomy of the

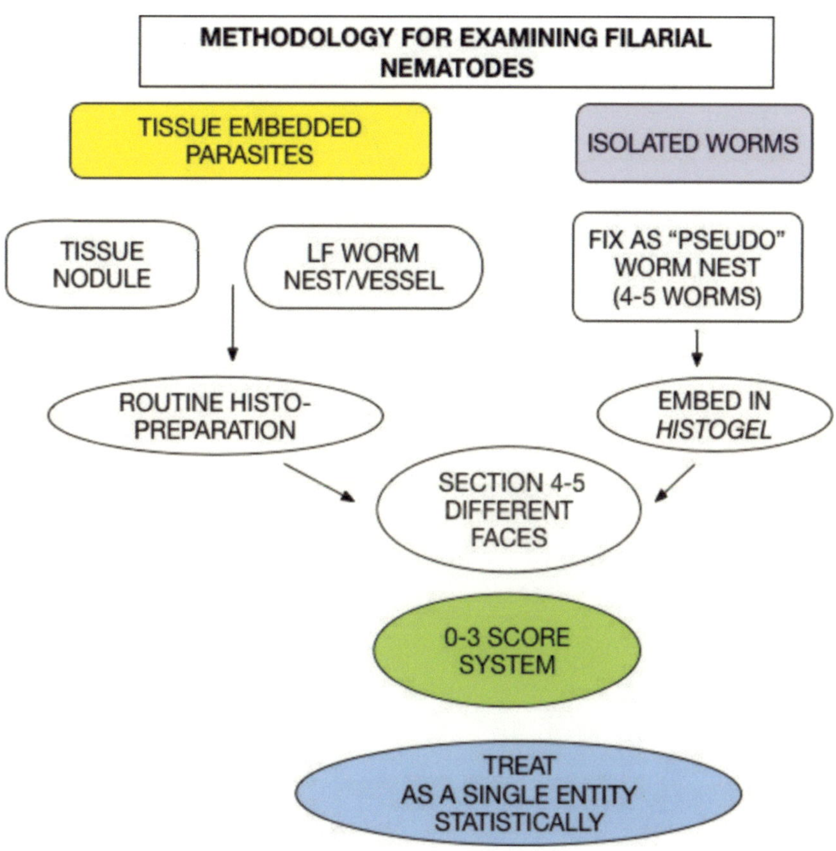

Figure 4. Stages of microfilariae developing in utero.

nematode before defining histologically changes that indicate degeneration and death. A summary of the major anatomical components that can be assessed is given in **Figure 3** and representative images in **Figure 5**. As already mentioned it is important to recognize that pathological changes within a degenerating worm can present differently at different points along the length of the organism, with changes occurring in one location and not in another within a single worm.

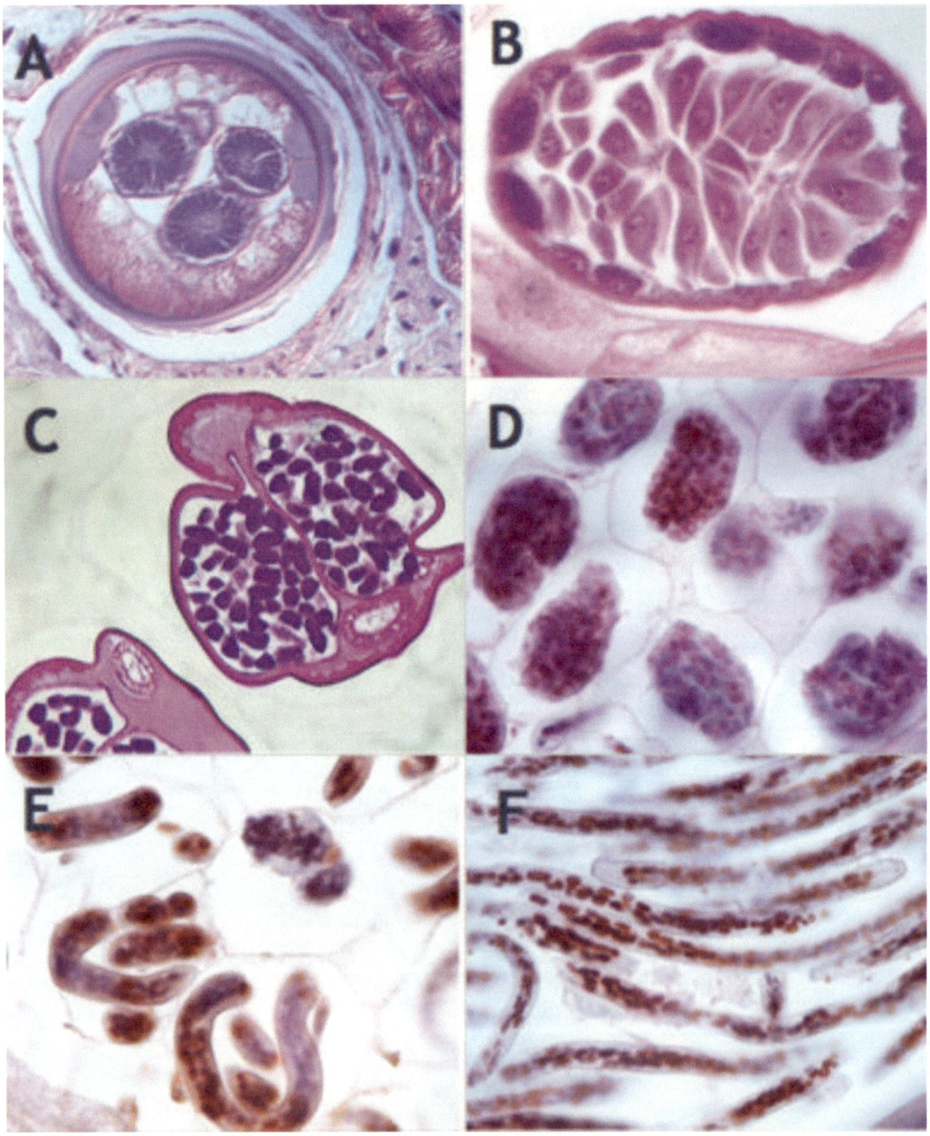

Figure 5. Normal components of adult female filarial nematodes. A. Ovaries of an onchocercal worm, B. Earliest stage of filarial ova, C. Morulae stages filling two uterine horns of a healthy female filarial worm, D. Mature morulae inside individual egg shells, E. Coiled microfilariae contained within egg shells, F. Fully stretched microfilariae ready for release from the uterus.

http://dx.doi.org/10.5772/intechopen.69512

Different ways of assessing the state of worms in histological sections have been used. A scoring system that has been developed and used successfully for the investigation of new chemotherapeutic agents [11, 12] and the type of degenerating forms seen in such studies shown in **Figure 6**. The use of a four-level score (0–3) for subjective assessments has been generally accepted in the realm of anatomical pathologists as minimizing, as much as possible, differences between observers and is a suitable formula for assessing nematodes.

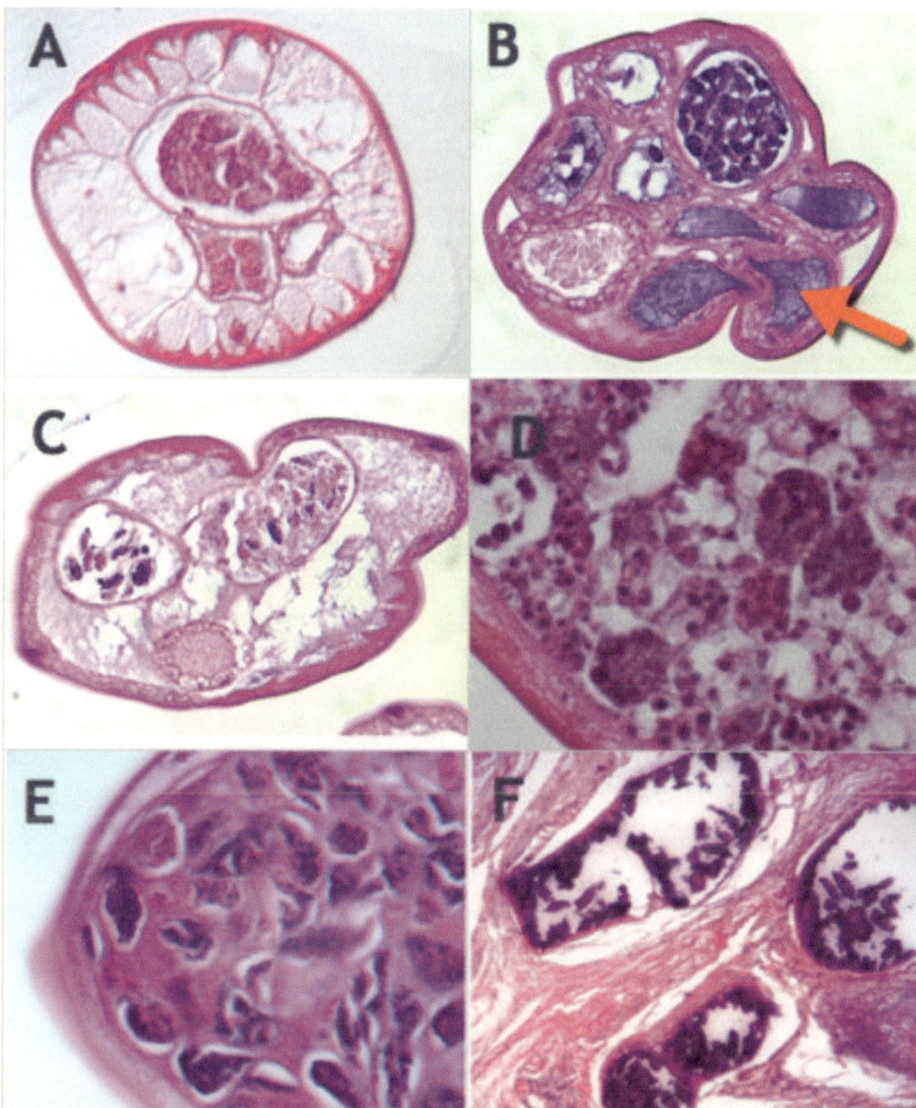

Figure 6. Examples of typical degenerative components of adult female filarial nematodes. A. Filarial nematode with damage to the body wall. B. Filarial nematode with damaged horns of the uterus with early calcification (blue staining of the uterine content), C. A degenerating worm with the morula stages unable to form. D. Disrupting early morulae forms E. Uterine horn of a damaged filarial worm containing many degenerating forms, F. Calcified casts of a dead filarial worm embedding in a chronic tissue response (nodule).

4.6. The assessment of *in vitro* worms

Much of what has been described for assessing parasites in *in vivo* situations applies to those parasites that have been obtained from culture systems. Here it is important to acknowledge that worms maintained *in vitro* are already in an unnatural environment and this can affect certain anatomical components more than others. The wall and cuticle of cultured worms often, even in the control samples, can have degenerative changes that are induced by this unusual environment. If worms have been isolated using tissue digestive methods before culturing then the changes due to the processing are consequently even more common.

A useful approach to preparing *in vitro* cultured worms for histology is to essentially prepare the worms as "nests" mimicking the natural situation seen in O*nchocerca* nodules, i.e. wrap the worms into a small artificial "balls", fix, embed and assess them as described above for the natural "nests" in onchocercal nodules (**Figure 3**). This collection of worms, optimally a minimum of 5 worms, is then regarded statistically as one entity (as are in vivo nodules). In cases where there is only a single worm available for a particular assay, then again, this worm should be coiled up into a small "ball" for processing; this approach allows for better statistical evaluation.

4.7. *In situ* markers of viability

The use of *in situ* markers is an important new approach being developed for assessing degenerative changes in nematodes but to date, there are still relatively few studies that address this issue in any great depth. One that has nevertheless been extensively described is the continuing presence of the required endosymbiont *Wolbachia*–usually identified by using labeled antibody markers against a primary antigen (WSP) of this bacterium. The presence of these organisms has been used as an indicator of the viability of the adult filarial worm. It must be recognized that this endosymbiont is not uniformly distributed along the worm and it is therefore relatively easy to be misled by only observing relatively few histological sections of the worm, many of which may naturally not actually contain this organism. It is also has been shown that MMP-2 and MMP-9 are two collagenases that are associated with *Wolbachia* in filariae, and a reduction in these two enzymes may reflect early damage to the adult worms [13].

There are several studies that have described several enzymes that appear to be present in filarial worms [14], and it is likely that specific enzymes will be identified soon whose presence could act as reliable indicators of worm viability. Biochemical approaches have been used to assess the viability of *in vitro* worms for many years–the formazan assay being commonly used [15–17]. Enzymes involved in general biochemical maintenance of nematodes [18], such as Nras have already been seen to provide some information as to the adult worms' integrity after chemotherapy [7].

4.8. Indirect markers

Although it is not a major purview of this discussion here to go into the wider area of laboratory and rapid test systems, it is nevertheless important to note that there is a considerable amount of experience over many years with the use of immunological markers, such as circulating antigens and host antibody responses for the diagnosis and epidemiological assessment of filarial infections, both in humans, dogs, and other animals [19]. In fact, with human lymphatic filariasis, the major diagnostic tool used in major public health control programs is a rapid diagnostic test for detecting circulating antigen in finger-prick sampled blood. In human onchocerciasis, the current approach is to use the presence of parasite-specific antibody (Ov16) to indicate the status of infection in an endemic community. The use of samples of urine and saliva for these assays has been attempted but with varying and unfortunately rather unuseful results to date.

There is an ever-increasing number of studies considering whether or not circulating specific products of parasites (e.g. protein microRNAs, etc) can reflect both the presence infection (in terms of the presence of different parasitic stages) or perhaps the load of infection (the intensity of infection). This is an area of research that is vital to the efforts to eliminate the major parasitic diseases across the world. It is likely that in the next few years specific circulating markers will be identified in blood, or hopefully (for ease of collection) in urine or in saliva. This would provide a more practical way to assesses populations in epidemiological studies and lead us more quickly to the global goal of eliminating nematodes for affected populations.

5. Discussion

There are still many aspects of measuring the viability of nematodes that need improving. A major challenge is to determine when a population of worms that have been subjected to an intervention, e.g. chemotherapy, an immune response, etc., and are on an irreversible pathway to death, and thus the parasite no longer can contribute to the infection in question. To achieve this, it is necessary at the level of the worm itself to understand what are the actual changes, or pathological events, within the worm's anatomy and biology that reflect permanent irreversible damage.

As described above it is relatively easy to detect alterations if they are physically obvious (e.g. calcified, broken and obviously damaged entities) but it is the interpretation of the less obvious changes in worms or the deceased levels of a marker indicator that is difficult; what level of damage is irreversible? Optimally it would be extremely useful to define a single change or a simple collection of changes that reflect permanent irreversible damage. In the case of filariae it is likely that the uterus (the biggest organ in the female) is a useful indicator site for detecting damage and defining permanent damage. The body wall is also an important target organ for this role but it is an organ that is easily artificially altered by many of the isolation techniques used in preparing the worm samples for studies, especially those for *in vitro* studies. Another reason for focusing on the uterus is that interruption of the reproductive capability is a major intervention goal for the three major filarial infections of humans and would be extremely valuable to the success of the current global elimination programs for these two infections.

The assessment approach used needs to be driven by the question being asked when deciding on the method and focus of any assessment. The complexity of the life cycle of nematodes necessitates carefully focusing investigations on stages or anatomical components that are likely to prove useful and provide practical information. The approaches used for assessment need in most cases to be closely associated with the programmatic question being addressed, and take into consideration the environmental situation at play; for example, the breaking of infection transmission or understanding the direct effect of a chemotherapeutic agent on the worm's reproductive capability. It is also important to distinguish between estimating parasite loads in an infected host and the measuring of direct effects on a parasite stage; although these two questions may be intimately linked they are not necessarily the same nor necessarily use the same method for assessment.

An obvious area of basic research that would greatly enhance the needs for developing better techniques for assessing parasite viability is advancing the knowledge of the basic physiological, biochemical and functional characteristics of nematodes and any species differences. Using *C. elegans* as the type model [20] is useful but filarial worms and other parasitic nematodes are considerably more complex and are likely to have different and unique characteristics. This kind of research is difficult to maintain in the present world where research funding is difficult to acquire, but nevertheless, the acquisition of more detailed information in this subject would undoubtedly be highly valuable. There is a tendency to interpret cell death, tissue damage and other pathological processes from the perspective of what we know about these processes in mammalian organisms and it would be extremely useful to know if there are similar or different processes occurring in metazoans.

Author details

Charles D. Mackenzie[1*], Ashley Behan-Braman[2], Joe Hauptman[2] and Timothy Geary[3]

*Address all correspondence to: tropmed@mac.com

1 Liverpool School of Tropical Medicine, Liverpool, UK

2 College of Veterinary Medicine, Michigan State University, East Lansing, Michigan, USA

3 McGill University, Montreal, Canada

References

[1] Shapiro-Ilan DI, Hazir S, Lete L. Viability and virulence of entomopathogenic nematodes exposed to ultraviolet radiation. Journal of Nematology. 2015;**47**(3):184-189. PMCID: PMC4612188

[2] Ferreira SR, Mendes AO, Bueno LL, de Araújo JV, Bartholomeu DC, Fujiwara RT. A new methodology for evaluation of nematode viability. BioMed Research International. 2015;**2015**: 879263. DOI: 10.1155/2015/879263

[3] Gyawali P, Sidhu JP, Ahmeda W, Jagals P, Tozea S. An approach to reduce false viability assessment of hookworm eggs with vital stains. Food and Waterborne Parasitology. 2016;**3**:9-12. http://dx.doi.org/10.1016/j.fawpar.2016.03.001

[4] Krose D, Zasada IA, Ingham RE. Comparison of Meldola's blue staining and hatching assay with potato root diffusate for assessment of *Globodera* sp. egg viability. Journal of Nematology. 2011;**43**(3-4):182-186

[5] James CE, Davey MW. A rapid colorimetric assay for the quantitation of the viability of free living larvae of nematodes in vitro. Parasitology Research. 2011;**101**:975-980

[6] Nutting CS, Eversole RR, Blair K, Specht S, Nutman TB, Klion AD, Wanji S, Boussinesq M, Mackenzie CD. Analysis of nematode motion using an improved light-scatter based system. PLoS Neglected Tropical Diseases. 2011;**9**(2):[e0003523]. DOI: 10.1371/journal.pntd.0003523

[7] Geary JF, Lovato R, Wanji S, Guderian R, O'Neill M, Specht S, Madrill N, Geary TG, Mackenzie CD. A histochemical study of the Nras/let-60 activity in untreated and ivermectin-treated adult *Onchocerca volvulus*. Parasites & Vectors. 2015;**8**:353. DOI: 10.1186/s13071-015-0947-6

[8] Schulz-Key H. The collagenase technique: How to isolate and examine adult *Onchocerca volvulus* for the evaluation of drug effects. Tropical Medicine and Parasitology. 1988;**39.** Suppl 4:423-440

[9] Maki J, Weinstein PP. Transplantation into jirds as a method of assessing the viability and reproductive integrity of adult *Acanthocheilonema viteae* from culture. Journal of Parasitology. 1991;**77**(5):749-754

[10] Peak E, Hoffmann KF. Cross-disciplinary approaches for measuring parasitic helminth viability and phenotype. Anais da Academia Brasileira de Ciências. Jun 2011;**83**(2):649-662

[11] O'Neill M, Geary JF, Agnew D, Mackenzie CD, Geary TG. In vitro flubendazole-induced damage to vital tissues in adult females of the filarial nematode Brugia malayi. International Journal of Parasitology: Drugs and Drug Resistance. 2015;**5**:135-140

[12] O'Neill M, Mansour A, DiCosty U, Geary J, Dzimianski M, McCall SD, McCall JW, Mackenzie CD, Geary TG. An in vitro/in vivo model to analyze the effects of flubendazole exposure on adult female *Brugia malayi*. PLOS Neglected Tropical Diseases. May 2016;**4**;10(5):e0004698. DOI: 10.1371/journal.pntd.0004698

[13] Gourley M, Mackenzie CD, Geary T, Lammie P, Lovato R, Eversole R. A role for collagenase in Wolbachia-filariid mutualism: in situ characterization of MMPs and *W. Pipientis* bacteria in the filarial parasite *Onchocerca volvulus*. Microbes and Infection in Press. 2017

[14] Bilslan E, Bean DM, Devaney E, Oliver SG. Yeast-based high throughput screens to identify novel compounds active against Brugia malayi. PLOS Neglected Tropical Diseases. 2016. DOI: 10.1371/journal.pntd.0004401

[15] Comley JC, Mike J. Rees MJ, Claire H. Turner CH, David C, Jenkins DC. Colorimetric quantitation of filarial viability. International Journal for Parasitology. 1989;**19**:77-83

[16] Comley JC, Claire H. Turner CH. Potential of a soluble tetrazolium/formazan assay for the evaluation of filarial viability. International Journal for Parasitology. 1990;**20**:251-255

[17] Strote G, Bokhof A, Comley JC. Viability of *Onchocerca volvulus* in vitro. Parasitology. 1993;**107**:175-182

[18] Misra S, Gupta J, Misra-Bhattacharya S. RNA interference mediated knockdown of Brugia malayi UDP Galactopyranose mutase severely affects parasite viability, embryogenesis and in vivo development of infective larvae. Parasites & Vectors. 2017;**10**(1):34. DOI: 10.1186/s13071-017-1967-1

[19] Hill DE, Forbes L, Kramer M, Gajadhar A, Gamble HR. Larval viability and serological response in horses with long-term *Trichinella spiralis* infection. Veterinary Parasitology. 2007;**146**(1-2): 107-116

[20] Mendoza AD, Woodruff TK, Wignall SM, O'Halloran TV. Zinc availability during germline development impacts embryo viability in *Caenorhabditis elegans*. Comparative Biochemistry and Physiology - Part C: Toxicology & Pharmacology. 2017;**191**:194-202. DOI: 10.1016/j.cbpc.2016.09.007

Chapter 7

The Impact of Plant-Parasitic Nematodes on Agriculture and Methods of Control

Gregory C. Bernard, Marceline Egnin and
Conrad Bonsi

Additional information is available at the end of the chapter

http://dx.doi.org/10.5772/intechopen.68958

Abstract

Plant-parasitic nematodes are costly burdens of crop production. Ubiquitous in nature, phytoparasitic nematodes are associated with nearly every important agricultural crop and represent a significant constraint on global food security. Root-knot nematodes (*Meloidogyne* spp.) cyst nematodes (*Heterodera* and *Globodera* spp.) and lesion nematodes (*Pratylenchus* spp.) rank at the top of list of the most economically and scientifically important species due to their intricate relationship with the host plants, wide host range, and the level of damage ensued by infection. Limitations on the use of chemical pesticides have brought increasing interest in studies on alternative methods of nematode control. Among these strategies of nonchemical nematode management is the identification and implementation of host resistance. In addition, nematode genes involved in parasitism represent key targets for the development of control through gene silencing methods such as RNA interference. Recently, transcriptome profiling analyses has been used to distinguish nematode resistant and susceptible genotypes and identify the specific molecular components and pathways triggered during the plant immune response to nematode invasion. This summary highlights the importance of plant-parasitic nematodes in agriculture and the molecular events involved in plant-nematode interactions.

Keywords: plant-parasitic nematodes, agriculture, crops, genetics, resistance, *Meloidogyne*

1. Introduction

Over millions of years, the association of plants and nematodes has resulted in the evolution of the plant-parasitic nematode. Widely distributed pathogens of vascular plants, enormous losses in yields have been attributed to the presence of nematodes. The intricate relationship between the parasitic nematode and plant has culminated in an "evolutionary arms race". Phyto-parasitic nematodes have evolved strategies to suppress host immune responses for the development of feeding sites. In turn, plants have developed specific molecules to recognize pathogens signaling the activation of immune responses. Declining use of chemical pesticides has brought great attention to research in alternative methods of nematode control. An effective strategy for nematode management involves the utilization and implementation of nematode-resistant cultivars into crop breeding programs. Currently, genetic sequencing analyses are widely utilized in the identification of molecular components of nematode parasitism and is also used to distinguish nematode-resistant and susceptible plant genotypes. These detailed analyses have significantly contributed to our overall understanding of the dynamic and complex nature of plant-nematode interactions.

2. Nematode morphology

Nematodes are a fascinating, biologically diverse group of organisms. Their ability to adapt to a wide variety of habitats including; marine, soil and aquatic, provides an evolutionary advantage for species longevity. Phylum Nematoda is largely distinguished by three major monophyletic groups including: Enoplia (marine), Dorylaimia (parasitic trichinellids and mermithids and Chromadoria (nematodes of various environments). Nematodes belong to the group Ecdysozoa, which comprises animals that can shed their cuticle. Over 30,000 species of round worms are found in Nematoda [1] typically ranging in size from 0.2 mm to over 6 m. Nematode body structure is relatively simple and characterized as limbless, cylindrical, and elongated. Essentially the body plan is a "tube within a tube", the inner tube or alimentary canal, consists of a digestive tract and gonad which are surrounded by an outer tube; a body wall containing a series of dorsal and ventral longitudinal muscles attached to the hypodermis. These muscles are activated by the dorsal and ventral nerves and their contractions allow for locomotion in sinusoidal waves. In plant-parasitic nematodes, a primary infection structure called a stylet is located at the anterior end of the nematode which is followed by an esophageal region that connects the stylet to the intestines. A typical tylenchoid esophagus consists of an anterior procorpus, a median bulb and the posterior basal bulb. The median bulb functions in the transfer of enzymes involved in primary infection and facilitates the movement of plant nutrients into the intestine. Inside of the exterior body wall lies the pseudocoelom, a unlined, pressurized, fluid-filled cavity formed directly from the blastula surrounding the gut cavity. The pseudocoelom is filled with fluid which provides turgor pressure for the entire body containing the internal organs and aides in the transfer of nutrients, oxygen and metabolic products. The excretory system is composed of four distinctive cells, an excretory pore cell, a duct cell, one canal cell, and a fused pair of gland cells. Nematodes are enclosed within an exoskeleton called a cuticle which is secreted by inner hypodermal cells, and is primarily composed of collagens, insoluble proteins (cuticlins), glycoproteins and lipids. The cuticle plays an important role in movement, environmental protection and growth and development [2]. The typical male reproductive structures include a testis, a seminal vesicle and a vas deferens leading to a cloaca, while the female reproductive system is tubular containing one or two ovaries, seminal receptacles, an uterus, ovijector and a vulva.

3. Evolution of plant-parasitic nematodes

Why do some nematodes become plant parasites? The dynamic association of nematode and plant host has resulted in plant parasitism which has evolved three times culminating in substantial benefits for nematode survival and development [3, 4]. An existing evolutionary hypothesis places the origins of these ancient microscopic roundworms around 400 million years before the explosion of animal phyla (pre-"Cambrian explosion") [5]. Evidence suggests the initial presence of plant-parasitic nematodes to have occurred around 235 BC [6] while the first described plant parasitic nematodes were reported by Needham who observed symptoms of galling in wheat [7]. An agriculturally important species of plant-parasitic nematodes called root-knot nematodes, were initially identified by Berkeley who observed the presence of galls on cucumber roots [8].

The plant-nematode association has resulted in the development of specific feeding structures and secretory products that are involved in host infection and nutrient absorption. Plant parasitic nematodes are specialized by the stylet and subventral and dorsal esophageal glands which are considered the most significant evolutionary adaptations for plant parasitism [4, 9]. Plant-parasitic nematodes utilize a hollow, needle-like, protrusible stylet to probe plant tissue and release an assortment of proteinaceous secretions from the subventral and dorsal glands which comprises the integrity of the host cell and allow for nematode entry. These glandular secretions induce cellular remodifications that are essential for development of a metabolically active feeding cell [10]. Among the secretory molecules are a group of carbohydrate-active enzymes. Since cellulose is the primary component of plant cell walls, cellulases (β-1,4-endoglucanases) are secreted to degrade the cell wall which allows nematode entry into host tissue. Genomic analyses of root-knot nematodes have revealed the presence of a suite of enzymes called CAZymes (cellulases, xylanases and other glycosyl hydrolase family members (GHFs)) [11]. Beta-1,4-endoglucanase genes have been isolated from plant-parasitic cyst nematodes with catalytic domains belonging to family 5 of the glycosyl hydrolases [12, 13].

Glycosyl hydrolase families G5 and G45 have been identified in plant-parasitic nematodes. Plant-parasitic nematode GH5 cellulases show closes homologies with bacterial G5s, which suggests an initial horizontal gene transfer of bacterial G5 cellulases into nematode genomes during the evolution of the plant-parasitic order Rhabditida (suborder Tylenchina) [14, 15]. G45 cellulases have been found in plant-parasitic nematode *Bursaphelenchus xylophilus* of the Aphelenchida order [16]. Phylogenetic analyses have shown similarities in gene structure between G45 sequences found in these nematodes and ascomycetous fungi which supports the hypothesis of a horizontal gene transfer event from fungi to nematodes [17].

Plant-parasitic nematodes differ in lifestyles. Some nematodes will invade the plant cells while others simply obtain nutrition externally. Ectoparasitic nematodes remain outside the host cells and feed on plant roots while endoparasitic nematodes establish residence within plant tissue. An example of ectoparasitic nematode is Xiphinema (California dagger nematode) which transmits the Grapevine fanleaf virus. The resulting viral infection causes tremendous economic losses in grapes worldwide [18]. Endoparasitic nematodes are further divided into migratory and sedentary groups. Migratory endoparasitic nematodes move within the root and remove cytoplasm killing the host cell while sedentary nematodes become immobile after the development of a feeding site within the host tissue [19]. Migratory endoparasitic nematodes of economic significance include *Pratylenchus* spp. (lesion nematode), *Radopholus* spp. (burrowing nematodes) and *Hirschmanniella* (rice root nematode).

4. The impact of plant-parasitic nematodes on crops

Plant-parasitic nematodes are a costly burden in agricultural crop production. Over 4100 species of plant-parasitic nematodes have been identified [20]. Collectively, they cause an estimated $80–$118 billion dollars per year in damage to crops [21, 22]. Encompassing 15% of all identified nematode species, the most economically important species directly target plant roots of major production crops and prevent water and nutrient uptake resulting in reduced agronomic performance, overall quality and yields. Nematodes in the order Tylenchida are pathogens of plants, invertebrates, and fungi and are considered the most important agricultural pests [22].

Of all the important plant-parasitic nematodes, the most successful species are the sedentary groups which establish a permanent feeding site within the plant host and obtain nutrients while completing their lifecycles. Sedentary nematodes have a natural advantage over their migratory relatives due to a fascinating and complex method of host cell transformation resulting in the development a sustainable feeding structure. Interestingly, with over 4000 described plant-parasitic nematodes, only a small amount produce significant economic losses in crops. In a survey conducted on a variety of crops in the U.S, the major genera of phytoparasitic nematodes reported to cause crop losses were *Heterodera, Hoplolaimus, Meloidogyne, Pratylenchus, Rotylenchulus,* and *Xiphinema* [23].

4.1. Wheat

Wheat (*Triticum aestivum*) is the most important cereal crop in the world. A staple food source for 40% of the world's population, approximately 758 million tons are produced globally [24]. Wheat yields are significantly decreased by the presence of cereal cyst nematodes (*Heterodera* spp.) in the *Heterodera avenae* group (*H. avenae, Heterodera filipjevi,* and *Heterodera latipons*) which also damage other important cereals including barley (*Hordeum vulgare*) and oat (*Avena sativa*). An estimated 3.4 million in profits are lost each year in U.S. wheat cultivating states Idaho, Oregon, and Washington [25]. In some wheat fields, the losses caused by *H. avenae* can range from 30 to 100% [26, 27]. In addition to cereal cyst nematodes, further losses of wheat are caused by root-lesion nematodes *Pratylenchus neglectus* and *Pratylenchus thornei,* and the seed gall or ear-cockle nematode, *Anguina tritici*. An inverse relationship between *H. avenae* and *P. neglectus* was shown on *P. neglectus* resistant and susceptible wheat cultivars infested with *H. avenae* [28] where a reduction in *P. neglectus* population densities was observed on both wheat genotypes. *Anguina tritici* is often a vector for *Rathayibacter tritici,* a Gram-positive soil bacterium which associates with *Clavibacter tritici* causing seed gall [29].

4.2. Rice

Rice (*Oryza sativa* L.) is a staple food crop for most of the world's population with an estimated 480 million tons currently produced [30]. Plant-parasitic nematodes rank as one of the most important soil borne pests of rice and may account for annual yield losses of 10–25% worldwide. Over 100 species of nematodes affect rice production. *Meloidogyne* spp. is distributed worldwide and are significant pathogens of rice and other crops cultivated in temperate and tropical areas [31]. One of the most important species of *Meloidogyne*, is *M. graminicola*, may reduce rice yields up to 80% [32]. Symptoms of infection manifests as hook shaped galls, stunting, decreased tiller numbers and poor growth and reproduction [33]. The rice root-nematode *Hirschmanniella oryzae*, i.e., rice root nematode (RRN), is commonly found in irrigated rice production systems [34]. Widely distributed, *H. oryzae* has been reported in Asian countries such as India, Pakistan, Bangladesh, Sri Lanka, Nepal, Thailand, Vietnam, Indonesia, the Philippines, China, Korea and Japan [35] and in the U.S states, Louisiana and Texas.

4.3. Maize

Maize (*Zea mays*) is grown largely throughout the world with three largest production in North America Asia and Europe [21]. Over 50 species that are known to parasitize corn in the globally however, the most devastating genera include the root knot nematodes, *Meloidogyne* spp., the root lesion nematodes, *Pratylenchus* spp. and the cyst nematodes, *Heterodera* spp. [21]. In the U.S., the most economically important species are the lesion nematodes (*Pratylenchus* spp.) and the corn cyst nematode (*Heterodera zeae*). In most cases, symptoms of infection caused by these nematodes include poor development and leaf chlorosis with minor galling [36]. The needle nematode *Longidorus breviannulatus* is associated with stunting in corn and may cause economic losses in yields up to 60% [37].

4.4. Potato

The potato (*Solanum tuberosum*) is a member of the Solanaceae family, and is considered the third most important crop in the world with total world potato production estimated at over 376 million tonnes in 2013 [38]. Cyst nematodes are prolific pathogens of potato causing dramatic losses in yields. *Globodera rostochiensis* and *Globodera pallida* originate from S. America and are known pests of other members of the Solanaceae family including tomatoes and woody nightshade [39]. These nematodes are classified as quarantine pests in a number of countries including the U.S. and an estimated £ 50m year in profits are lost each year in the U.K. [40]. Other major plant-parasitic nematodes of potato include root-knot nematodes (*Meloidogyne* spp.), and the stem nematode *Ditylenchus destructor*. Among the four species of root-knot nematodes that affect potato production in the U.S., the Columbian root-knot nematode (*Meloidogyne chitwoodii*) is considered the most important species [41]. In addition to potato, sweetpotato (Ipomoea *batatas* L. Lam) is a major host for *D. destructor*, up to 100% yield losses have occurred in major production regions including the top producer China [42, 43]

4.5. Sweetpotato

The sweetpotato [*Ipomoea. batatas* (L) LAM] has been regarded as a plant of great significance throughout human history. Its cultivation dates to the prehistoric era, and it has been grown continuously as a staple food source. Global productions of sweetpotato is estimated at 105 million metric tons [44]. Currently, the sixth most important food crop, sweetpotato production has improved the economic status for communities throughout the world particularly in developing nations where it ranks as the fifth most important crop [44]. Approximately 10.2% of sweetpotato yields are lost each year due to the presence of plant-parasitic nematodes [20]. Root-knot nematodes (RKNs) are significant pests of sweetpotato causing symptoms of infection which include: stunted plant growth, yellowing of leaves, abnormal flower production, and gall production on roots leading to decreased nutrient and water absorption and necrosis and cracking on fleshy storage roots. Due to the economic importance of the storage root, root cracking is a primary concern for producers. Successful sweetpotato root-knot nematode resistant breeding programs involve the determination of resistance genes. Nematode resistance is governed by genotype [45] and is primarily quantitative [46]; therefore, the identification of genetic markers associated with root-knot nematode resistance requires broad scale molecular studies.

4.6. Root-knot nematodes

In a recent survey, the top 10 most important genera of parasitic nematodes in molecular plant pathology were ranked based on scientific and economic importance [47]. Ranked at the top of the list are root-knot nematodes (*Meloidogyne* spp.). The root-knot nematode (*Meloidogyne* spp.) comprises over 100 species, with *Meloidogyne javanica, Meloidogyne arenaria, Meloidogyne hapla,* and *Meloidogyne incognita* representing the most devastating threat to agricultural crop production [48]. The *Meloidogyne* spp. are globally distributed, have enormous host range and develop dynamic disease complexes with fungal species and bacteria which may exacerbate disease incidences in cultivated plants. The lifecycle of *Meloidogyne* spp. involves four developmental stages including larval stage 1 (within the egg), larval stage 2 (migratory), larval stage juvenile 3 (sedentary), larval stage 4 (sedentary) and adult stage (sedentary). Under favorable environmental conditions, first stage moulting to J1 larval stage within the egg occurs resulting in hatching, with or without the presence of a chemical stimulus. Infective second-stage juveniles (J2s) are often attracted to root exudates and migrate to root tips where they infiltrate behind the root cap at the elongation zone. Root knot nematodes attenuate plant cells by stylet thrusting and secrete cell wall degrading enzymes to separate the middle lamella during intercellular migration through root cortex cells as they target the undifferentiated procambium cells of the vascular cylinder. During later stages in primary infection, dorsal gland activity increases to promote shuttling of secretory granules to the stylet where proteinaceous secretions are released in the development of the primary feeding site—the giant cell [49]. The multi-nucleated giant cell is a result of nematode-induced endoreduplication within the host cell in the absence of cytokinesis. Cellular ingrowths arise to sequester solutes from the xylem [50] further enhancing nutrient availability. J2 larvae moult into larval stage 3 (J3) during the initial intake of plant nutrients from giant cells. Additional moulting occurs resulting into the J4 and final adult stage. Further reproductive development in females results in the characteristic "apple" shape associated with the Greek nomenclature *Meloidogyne*. The lifecycle completes when eggs are released into the soil from the gelatinous egg matrix formed on epidermal root tissue. Root-knot nematode infection is typically characterized by stunted growth, wilting, root galling and abnormalities in root formation.

4.7. Cyst nematodes

Cyst forming nematodes, or cyst nematodes, (*Heterodera* and *Globodera* spp.) rank second to root-knot nematode in agricultural and economic importance. The biology of cyst nematodes is similar to that of root-knot nematodes where J2 larvae infect the host and develop to adult stages within host tissue. In contrast, to root-knot nematode reproduction where eggs are deposited into a gelatinous matrix on root systems, eggs produced by cyst nematodes are preserved within the body of the female and are protected after her death until hatching under favorable conditions. Cyst nematodes enter root tips and induce specialized feeding structures in the infected plant roots called syncytia via esophageal gland secretions released by the stylet [51]. These secretions promote cell wall degradation and protoplast fusion of numerous adjacent cells to form the syncytium [52]. In agriculture, the most significant cyst nematode species are the potato cyst nematodes *Globodera rostochiensis* and *G. pallida*, the soybean cyst nematode (*Heterodera glycines*) and cereal cyst nematodes (CCNs) (including *Heterodera avenae* and *H. filipjevi*. In the U.S., losses due to *H. glycines* is estimated at 1.286 billion [53]. *Globodera pallida* originated in South America and is now widely distributed in 55 countries. Yield losses of potato due to *G. pallida* range from 50 to 80% in heavily infested soils [54]. Although the beet cyst nematode, *Heterodera schachtii*, is a primary pathogen of sugar beets, it can parasitize plant species in 23 different plant families with losses of 30% in the families of *Chenopodiaceae* [55, 56].

4.8. Lesion nematodes

Ranked third among the most damaging nematodes in agriculture [57], approximately 70 species of root-lesion nematodes (*Pratylenchus* spp.) are distributed worldwide with a host range of nearly 400 plant species [57]. Among *Pratylenchus* spp., *P. thornei* is associated with yield reductions in wheat by as much as 85% in Australia, 70% in Israel, 50% in Oregon and 37% in Mexico [58]. Lesion nematodes are migratory, feeding mainly in the root cortex and may enter vascular tissues obtaining nutrients. Infection typically results in lesion formation and necrosis on roots with aboveground symptoms of chlorosis as well as reductions in leaf number and size [58, 59]. Host tissue injury resulting from infection may represent areas for secondary infection from other pathogens. Recently two new species of root-lesion nematodes (*Pratylenchus. kumamotoensis, Pratylenchus. pseudocoffeae*) were identified in Korea by morphometric and molecular analyses of internal transcribed spacer (ITS) and ribosomal DNA [60].

4.9. Burrowing nematode

The burrowing nematode, *Radopholus similis* [(Cobb, 1893) Thorne, 1949] is a migratory plant parasitic nematode, listed as a quarantine plant pest worldwide [61]. Over 250 plant species serve as hosts for *R. similis* where it causes severe economic losses in yields. *R. similis* damages banana, citrus, pepper, coffee and other agronomic and horticultural crops and is considered the most important phytopathogenic nematode in banana-growing areas [62]. Effective control of *R. similis* remains problematic worldwide, and effective approaches must be identified and implemented. *Radopholus* Calreticulin (CRT) is a Ca^{2+}-binding protein that plays key roles in parasitism and represents a candidate target for controlling *R. similis. R. similis* CRT (*Rs-CST*) is expressed in the esophageal, reproductive and gastrointestinal regions as well as the eggs. Using plant-mediated RNA interference, *Rs-CRT* expression was significantly inhibited in the nematodes, and enhanced resistance was demonstrated in transgenic tomato plants [63]. In a bioassay-based study, phenylphenalenones extracted from Musa spp. showed anti-nematode effects on *R. similis* which was demonstrated by nematode motility inhibition [64].

5. Nematode parasitism genes

Nematode parasitism is conferred by the actions of a variety of genes that are upregulated during host infection. In an earlier review, a comprehensive discussion highlighted the structure, origin and functions of nematode parasitism genes and further supported the acquisition of parasitism genes through horizontal transfer from bacteria [49]. Since parasitism genes are usually required for infection, they represent important targets for the development of control measures. Parasitism genes often encode for effectors which are proteins or chemicals that elicit an immune response and/or trigger changes in the host cell architecture [51]. Recently two effector genes (*MhTTL2* and *Mh265*) were identified in the root-knot nematode *M. hapla* and were shown to be upregulated during primary infection [65]. *MhTTL2* encodes for a secreted protein bearing a transthyretin-like protein domain and is expressed in the amphids, with a potential role in the nervous system while *Mh265* is expressed in subventral glands. Nematode effectors including expansin, β-1,4-endoglucanase and polygalacturonase are released during primary infection and feeding site development. In plants, expansin proteins are secreted during growth processes to allow for cell enlargement [66]. Nematodes are believed to cause differential expressions of plant genes encoding cell wall modifying proteins including expansins [67] quite possibly to mimic endogenous expansin production during feeding site development. HaEXPB2, a predicted expansin-like protein found in cereal cyst nematode *Heterodera avenae* was associated with cell death in tobacco plants [68]. During primary infection of tobacco, *HaEXPB2* gene expression was localized in subventral glands of J2 nematodes and was later found in the cell wall. Silencing of *HaEXPB2* by RNA interference was associated with reduced nematode infectivity. Transcriptome sequencing analyses of early stage *H. avenae* juveniles has revealed a variety of potential effectors including plant cell wall-modifying proteins and homologues of secreted proteins involved in the detoxification of reactive oxygen species (ROS) including: peroxiredoxin, glutathione peroxidase, glutathione-S-transferase [69]. ROS release is associated with onset of plant defense signaling. New evidence suggests that root-knot nematodes may utilize plant peroxidase to reduce ROS levels and parasitize plants bearing the *Mi-1* root-knot nematode resistance gene [70]. In plants, pathogens may trigger a hypersensitive response which involves programmed

http://dx.doi.org/10.5772/intechopen.68958

cell death (a form of apoptosis) in the site of infection to prevent pathogen colonization. Apoptosis regulator BAX (BCL-2 protein 4) is a member of the Bcl-2 family of proteins found in plants and animals [71]. Two secretory effector candidate genes (No. 5, No. 100) identified by transcriptome profiling in *Meloidogyne enterolobii* suppressed BAX-induced programmed cell death suggesting their roles as plant immune modulators for nematode infection [72]. The SPRY (SPla and the RYanodine Receptor) protein domain is most likely a scaffold for mediating protein-protein interactions [73]. SPRY effectors from *Globedera* spp. was shown to suppress the plant defense responses [74].

6. Molecular basis of nematode resistance

The development of a resistance response may encompass a variety of physiological outcomes including: minor or complete absence of galling, differences in the degree of necrosis, the inability of the nematode to establish a permanent feeding site, and a decrease in female fecundity or egg output. To date, the majority of plant-parasitic nematode resistance genes bear the characteristic NBS-LRR (Nucleotide binding site—Leucine Rich Repeat) domains. These include the *Mi-1* gene from *Solanum peruvianum* (formerly *Lycopersicon peruvianum*) [75], *Hs1*$^{pro\text{-}1}$ from sugar beet [76] and *Gpa2* and *Gro1-4* from potato [77, 78].

Resistance to *Meloidogyne* in commercial resistant tomato cultivars (*Lycopersicon esculentum*) was originally identified in its wild relative *L. peruvianum* Mill. [79] followed by introgression of resistance into commercial breeding lines through backcrossing [80]. Several root-knot resistance gene homologues have been identified in tomato. *Mi-1.2* (referred to as *Mi-1*) confers resistance to multiple species of root-knot nematodes, [75] the potato aphid, *Macrosiphum euphoribiae* [81] and the whitefly, *Bemisia tabaci* [82]. *Rme1* is considered a potential component of the *Mi-1*-mediated signaling pathway as studies have indicated tomato *Rme1* mutants lack resistance to nematodes and whiteflies [66]. Molecular changes in *Rme1* protein conformation due to the presence of pathogens, may be recognized by *Mi-1.1* which signals the hypersensitive response in the "guard hypothesis" [83]. In carrots, inherited dominance of two root-knot nematode resistance genes *Mj1* [84] and *Mj2* [85] conferred resistance to *M. javanica*. The *RMIa* gene located in a subtelomeric position 300 kb physical distance between AMPP117 and AMPP116 markers and is associated with *M. incognita* resistance in peach (*Prunus* spp.) [86]. The Myrobalam plum (*Prunus cerasifera*) harbors dominant alleles (*Ma1*, *Ma2*, and *Ma3*) of a single gene *Ma*, a TIR-NBS-LRR class resistance gene, which confers broad spectrum resistance to multiple *Meloidogyne* spp. [87]. Using polymorphic sequencing analyses and genetic linkage mapping (RFLP, SSR) the *Ma* loci was precisely identified in the Myrobalan plum linkage group 7, while in a Japanese plum variety, a *Rjap* gene was localized at the same position in co-segregation with SSR markers previously associated with root-knot nematode resistance [88]. In sweetpotato, 275 candidate resistance gene analogs have been identified by degenerate PCR and molecular mining [89]. Plant-parasitic nematodes have been shown to manipulate host gene expression, therefore the identification of differential expression patterns of transcript levels for defense-related genes is a critical component in the determination of molecular factors of root-knot nematode resistance. Traditional identification of root-knot nematode resistance has involved the use of bulk segregant analysis [90] to map out qualitative traits between pooled plant genomes. Bulk segregant analysis has been used in tandem with random amplified polymorphic DNA assays to identify molecular markers at specific loci associated with root knot resistance in sweetpotato where genotypes are often isogenic [91]. Polymorphic events in resistance genes that confer effector recognition has been demonstrated in *Arabidopsis* resulting in a bifurcation that distinguishes resistant and susceptible allele clades [92].

Genome-wide expression profiling analyses using next-generation sequencing technologies are often employed in the analysis of host-nematode interactions. The resultant data from global transcriptome assays are used to target genetic traits associated with plant immune responses in response to various pathogens and to distinguish plant genotypes for resistance or susceptibility to certain diseases. Our general understanding of discreet molecular events involved in compatible (susceptible) and incompatible (resistant) plant-nematode interactions is limited in comparison to other significant host-pathogen associations. Recently, RNA-Sequencing has been frequently used in plant pathological studies to profile gene expression patterns in host plants and pathogens [93, 94]. Differential genetic expression profiles of many specific genes involved in plant immune responses has been shown in resistant and susceptible plants challenged by root-knot nematodes [48, 95]. The identification of novel defense-related transcripts and the elucidation of pathways involved in plant immune responses to nematodes have been recorded for important economic crops including cotton [96], rice [97], and soybean [98]. Transcriptome profiling of resistant and susceptible tobacco varieties infected with root-knot nematodes has shown differential expression patterns among genes involved in cell wall modification, auxin production and oxidative stress [99].

6.1. Plant immune responses

Due to their immobile lifestyle, plants have developed sophisticated molecular strategies to prevent pathogen invasion [100]. Plant defense has been characterized as a two- prong approach. In incompatible (resistant) plant-pathogen interactions, the presence of microbial/pathogen/-associated molecular patterns (M/PAMPs) including: toxins, glycoproteins, carbohydrates, fatty acids and proteins can trigger the upregulation of a network of host genes and corresponding proteins involved in an innate response termed pathogen-triggered immunity (PTI). Plant pathogens have evolved specialized effector molecules to suppress this first line of defense leading to effector-trigged susceptibility (ETS). In turn, plants have developed resistance genes which recognize specific effectors triggering a more robust defense response characterized as effector-triggered immunity (ETI). A hallmark of ETI is a hypersensitive cell death response (HR) at the infection site which prevents pathogen colonization [101].

6.2. Reactive oxygen species and antioxidant production

During plant metabolic processes, the accumulation of reactive oxygen species (ROS) by-products including superoxide anion (O_2^-), hydrogen peroxide (H_2O_2), singlet oxygen ($^1O_2$)

and hydroxyl radicals (^{-}OH) is often continuous, as these highly reactive molecules are localized to various cellular compartments. ROS are primarily generated by NADPH oxidases and superoxide dismutases and production is associated with numerous abiotic and biotic stress responses. Activation of ROS was shown to be critical during the defense response to root-knot nematode invasion [102]. ROS accumulation is toxic to nematodes and can often lead to induced oxidative destruction of infected cells during the hypersensitive response, to prohibit pathogen colonization. Increased ROS production is often correlated with the activation of antioxidant gene expression. These oxidative/reduction reactions must be tightly regulated to eliminate inadvertent plant tissue damage. Antioxidant enzymes including peroxidases are primarily responsible for the maintenance of a steady-state ROS level however, certain classes of peroxidases act as producers of ROS depending on the cyclic (catalytic or the hydroxylic) nature of the enzyme. ROS- producing Class III peroxidase genes were upregulated during an incompatible reaction in *H. avenae*-resistant wheat cultivars [103]. Peroxidase reduces H_2O_2 levels via H_2O_2-dependent polymerization of hydroxycinnamyl alcohols which promotes defense responses including lignin synthesis and cell-wall reinforcement by the cross-linkage of cell wall proteins [104]. Higher induction of peroxidase groups was observed in resistant plant species during *H. avenae* and *M. incognita* infection [105].

6.3. Pathogenesis-related proteins

Presently, 17 families of pathogenesis-related (PR) proteins have been identified based primarily on their enzyme function, activity and amino acid sequence homologies [106]. The PR family are characterized as plant allergens inclusive of an assortment of proteins such as: b-1,3 glucanases, chitinases, proteinase inhibitors, defensins, ribonucleases and thionins. PR gene expression is often induced by ethylene, salicylic acid, jasmonic acid, xylanase, and systemin signaling pathways. The molecular functions of PR proteins are often species specific with great diversity in the mode of action and structure between protein groups. Most PRs possess antifungal, antiviral, antibacterial and insecticidal activity and are primarily involved in plant developmental processes and environmental stress responses. PR proteins were initially reported in tobacco leaves during a hypersensitive response to the tobacco mosaic virus (TMV) [107, 108] and have been induced in response a wide variety of pathogens including nematodes. During nematode infections, PR transcripts may accumulate in high concentrations and are associated with the long distance immune response termed systemic acquired resistance (SAR) [109]. Increased expression of *PR-1*(P4) transcripts was observed at 3 days' post-infection in the *G. rostochiensis*-infected resistant plants compared with the uninoculated controls [110].

6.4. Callose deposition

Cell wall modifications often occur during plant-pathogen interactions which are demonstrated by the deposition of cell wall appositions leading to the development of papillae. Structural components associated with papillae formation are: callose, phenolics including lignin, phenolic conjugates such as phenolic–polyamines, reactive oxygen species, peroxidases, cell wall structural proteins (arabinogalactan proteins and hydroxyproline-rich glycoproteins) and cell wall polymers (pectin and xyloglucans). Callose (beta-1-3-glucan) deposition, lignification and suberization are plant developmental processes further associated with the restriction of systemic pathogen movement during PTI. Defense-associated cell wall strengthening through lignin and callose synthesis is signaled by cell wall degradation in a feedback mechanism which occurs in response to pathogens [111]. In addition to promoting declines in localized microbial populations, callose deposition also prevents the translocation of PTI-suppressive effectors. Interestingly, the cuticular chitin derivatives of plant-parasitic nematodes may activate the innate immune response. Although the cuticle is generally believed to be devoid of chitin, it is possible that chitin derivatives or chitin previously deposited in the stylet are recognized by the host which activates callose deposition at the site of penetration. The overexpression of the ethylene response transcription factor RAP2.6 in *Arabidopsis* enhanced plant basal resistance to *H. schachtii* [112]. Increased expression of jasmonic acid-related genes and callose deposition were observed at nematode infection sites.

7. WRKY transcription factors

WRKY transcription factors are transcriptional regulators of many developmental processes in plants and are associated with abiotic and biotic stress responses. The WRKY domain is almost exclusive to plants characterized by a highly-conserved core WRKYGQK motif and a zinc finger region. The critical role of WRKY transcription factors (WRKY TFs) in plant defense responses has been well documented [113, 114]. Their ability to bind to pathogen responsive cis acting W-box promoter elements in *PR1* genes is indicative of their role in plant immunity [113]. *Arabidopsis WRKY72* was reported to have a significant contribution to *Mi-1*-mediated defense against RKNs, potato aphids [114] and oomycete pathogen *Hyaloperonospora arabidopsidis* the causal agent of downy mildew [115]. *WRKY* gene expression is altered during plant-parasitic nematode interactions. The development of cyst nematode *H. schachtii* feeding site (syncytia) involves the up-regulation of WRKY23 [116]. Conversely, endogenous *WRKY33* gene expression levels were strongly downregulated in syncytia formed in *Arabidopsis* roots, while plants overexpressing *WRKY33* showed a 20–30% reduction in the presence of female nematodes [117] a possible indication of its role in plant defense.

7.1. Calreticulin proteins

In animals, endoplasmic reticulum (ER) localized calreticulin proteins are integral components in calcium homeostasis as well as protein folding and are involved in other significant cellular functions [118]. Ubiquitously expressed in plants, calreticulin performs similar functions to its animal counterpart despite 50% differences in amino acid sequence homology. Plant calreticulin is described as a molecular calcium-binding chaperone that promotes protein folding, calcium signaling and homeostasis, and oligomeric assembly in a calreticulin/calnexin cycle. Calreticulin may interact with a majority of monoglucosylated glycoproteins synthesized in the ER, while certain isoforms have been associated with the expression and quality control of the elongation factor Tu receptor-like protein kinase (EFR) [119] an important event in M/PAMP-triggered immune responses. The significance of calreticulin isoform-3 (*AtCRT-3*) function through gene deletion was identified in *Arabidopsis* plants [120]. Plant transformants with repressed *AtCRT*-3 gene activity were impaired in perception of M/PAMP-associated efl-18 and deficient in EFR protein expression and anthocyanin content. Furthermore, they concluded that AtCRT-3 may be involved in the unfolding and activation of EFR based on its primary molecular function and recognition of EFR N-glycosyl binding sites. Recently, studies have shown that root-knot nematodes secrete calreticulin, which plays an important role in infection [121].

7.2. Plant proteinase inhibitors

Plants utilize an arsenal of defensive mechanisms to evade infection from nematodes. One important strategy involves limiting nematode feeding capabilities. Plant proteinase inhibitors are involved in many physiological processes including protein turnover and proteolysis during metabolism however; other evidence has supported an alternative role in defense against plant pathogens [122]. Plant proteinase inhibitors degrade nematode proteases preventing the breakdown of food material which reduces nutrient absorption in the nematode. As early as 1947, the idea of proteinaceous protease inhibitors was formulated as Mickel and Standish observed differences in larval development on soybean cultivars [123]. The applicability of proteinase-inhibitors in nematode resistance was initially demonstrated in transgenic potato expressing a serine proteinase-inhibitor cowpea trypsin inhibitor (CpTI) [124]. CpTI expression directly influenced the sexual fate of *G. pallida* toward a higher ratio of smaller males with reduced damage observed on roots. Out of the four major classes of plant proteinases inhibitors (cysteine, serine, aspartic, metallo-proteinases) cysteine and serine proteinase inhibitors have gained considerable interest as effective defense molecules nematodes due to their specificity in the degradation of the major digestive enzymes (proteases) in plant-parasitic nematodes [125].The effectiveness of proteinase inhibitors can be attributed to its small size, which benefits its inclusion with nutrient molecules absorbed by some plant-parasitic nematodes. In tomato, overexpression of phytocystatin gene, *CeCPI* isolated from taro (*Colocasia esculenta*) showed enhanced resistance to root-knot nematodes demonstrated by reduced galling and an influence on sex determination [126]. In sweetpotato, sporamin which is classified as a Kunitz-type trypsin inhibitor, accounts for 60–80% of total soluble protein. Sporamin is constitutively expressed in the tuberous root in comparison to in the stem or leaves and is expressed systemically in response to wounding and other abiotic stresses [127]. In previous studies, three forms of sweetpotato sporamin showed strong trypsin inhibitory activity *invitro* [128]. Additional research has resulted in the identification of sporamin-mediated resistance to cyst nematodes [129]. Decreased nematode development correlated with trypsin inhibitor activity of sporamin which was the critical factor for inhibition of growth and development of cyst nematodes on sugar beet roots. Plant genotypes that produce high sporamin levels may have a selective advantage in defense to plant-parasitic nematodes.

7.3. Plant hormones

The roles of plant developmental hormones, ethylene, jasmonic acid and salicylic acid have been well established during plant immunity [130, 131]. Jasmonic acid (JA) and ethylene (ET) signaling pathways work synergistically while the salicylic acid (SA) pathway is antagonistic to JA/ET pathways [132]. In a prior study, exogenous ethyhlene (ethephon) and jasmonic acid (methyl jasmonate) application triggered the induction of PR proteins and the activation of systemic defense against root-knot nematodes on rice [133] These findings suggest a critical role of an active intact jasmonic acid pathway during the activation of systemically induced resistance. The combination of exogenous jasmonic acid and biogenic elicitor arachidonic acid, decreased galling on tomato roots two-fold in comparison to controls [134]. The role of salicylic acid has been well documented in the efficacy of host resistance to root-knot nematodes. Pathogenesis-related protein expression was associated with salicylic acid-dependent systemic required resistance in tomatoes pretreated with salicylic acid under root-knot nematode challenge [109]. Expression of a *NahG* which encodes for an enzyme that degrades salicylic acid to catechol, reduced *Mi-1* gene- mediated root-knot nematode resistance in transgenic tomatoes [135].

8. Disease management of plant-parasitic nematodes

8.1. Cultural control

For many years, crop rotation and cover cropping are often utilized in integrated pest management protocols to reduce plant-parasitic nematode incidence and replenish soil nutrient levels. Soil nematode levels have been effectively decreased by rotational cultivation of non-host cultivars however, the wide host range of *Meloidogyne spp.* often diminishes the effectiveness of crop rotation [136]. Planting corn as a rotational crop has been shown to reduce northern root-knot nematode (*M. hapla*) incidence however; population densities of other *Meloidogyne spp.* may increase with persistent cultivation. Plant species with resistance to mixed *Meloidogyne* populations have been identified. Leguminous cover crops *Mucuna pruriens* L., and *Crotalaria spectabilis* showed multiple resistance to three species of root-knot nematodes (*Meloidogyne arenaria, M. incognita, M. javanica*) [137]. In certain cases, the very nature of crop production may suppress the magnitude of infection. Rice is cultivated under flooding conditions which does not favor the nematode lifestyle. In Taiwan, crop rotations with rice or taro combined with cultural control methods including flooding and bare fallowing was shown to decrease nematode soil populations and increase strawberry yields [138].

8.2. Plant extracts

Plant extracts often contain a myriad of compounds which demonstrate nematode suppressive properties. Ethanolic extracts of *Azadirachta indica* (neem), *Withania somnifera* (ashwagandha), *Tagetes erecta* (marigold) and *Eucalyptus citriodora* (eucalyptus) were reported to show nematicidial activity against *Meloidogyne incognita, Helicotylenchus multicinctus* and *Hoplolaimus* which was comparable to chemical nematicide controls [139]. In other reports, increased plant growth and development were shown in plants propagated with the addition of a variety of extracts. Root-knot nematode egg hatch and larval development was dramatically reduced by leaf extracts from *Hunteria umbellata* and *Mallotus oppositifolius* which coincided with

http://dx.doi.org/10.5772/intechopen.68958

increased growth of cashew seedlings [140]. Plant height, fruit production and weights of *M. incognita*-infected tomato were significantly increased by the addition of ethanol extracts from *Azadirachta indica* leaves, *Capsicum annuum* fruits, *Zingiber officinale* rhizomes and *Parkia biglobosa* seeds in comparison to non-treated controls [141].

8.3. Biological control

With increasing demands in organic agriculture and concerns for environmental welfare, the use of chemical pesticides has decreased. Alternative means of pest management such as the use of biological controls are of great interest for crop producers. The efficacy of nematophagous bacteria and fungi in the control some nematode pests, including cyst and root-knot nematodes has been well-documented [142, 143]. Parasitic bacteria of *Pasteuria spp.* have been reported to infect 323 nematode species including both plant-parasitic nematodes and free-living nematodes [144]. Three methods of application for *P. penetrans* were evaluated for nematode control including seed, transplant, and post-plant treatments [145]. In greenhouse studies involving cucumber, all three *Pasteuria* treatments were shown to reduce galling caused by *M. incognita* as well as soil nematode numbers and nematode reproduction. In other reports, *M. incognita* suppression was observed in field soil treated with *P. penetrans* in comparison to untreated soil [146]. Other genera of bacteria including *Bacillus* spp. have shown great promise in nematode management. *B. cereus* strain S2 treatment resulted in a mortality of 90.96% to *M. incognita* [147]. *B. firmus* YBf-10 exhibited nematicidal activity against *M. incognita*, which was clearly demonstrated by an inhibition of egg hatch and motility [148]. Nematophagous fungi *Pochonia chlamydosporia* has potential as a biological control agent for *M. incognita* in vegetable crops. Along with crop rotational methods, *P. chlamydosporia* was shown to reduce nematode levels in soil previously used for root-knot nematode susceptible tomato [149]. Nematophagous fungal products including chitinases show great potential for the development of biopesticides. Certain root-knot nematode species have transparent protective chitin-containing shells. Purified chitinase LPCHI1 from *Lecanicillium psalliotae* was shown to degrade *M. incognita* eggs [150].

8.4. Host resistance

Chemical nematicides are often used in the management of root-knot nematodes however; EPA restrictions in some soil fumigants due to increased environmental toxicity coupled with the expensive costs associated new nematicide development limit their availability. The very nature of these mammalian pesticides poses a significant risk to humans. Plant-parasitic nematodes often reside in plant tissue which makes soil delivery applications of the chemical challenging. The incorporation of plant varieties that harbor multiple resistance to an array of plant pathogens is an attractive and practical approach for plant breeders. However, the conserved use of specific genotypes of disease resistant cultivars may contribute to increased pathogen aggressiveness resulting in epiphytotic conditions; therefore the identification of additional resistant varieties becomes increasingly necessary for long term control. For many years crops have been artificially selected for their inherent disease-resistant properties through phenotypic screenings and genetic analyses. Nematode-resistant genes found in gene pools of a variety of plant species have been introgressed into the genomes of economically important crops with natural susceptibility through transgenic technologies such as agrobacterium-mediated transformation [151, 152].

Plants synthesize and release an array of volatile organic compounds in response to damage. Plant terpenes/terpenoids are secondary metabolites produced by terpene synthases in plants and are involved plant survival and biotic and abiotic stress responses. Functional characterization of one member of the soybean TPS gene family, designated GmAFS suggested an anti-nematode role [153]. Transgenic hairy roots overexpressing GmAFS were generated in an *H. avenae*-susceptible soybean line. Plants showed significantly higher resistance to *H. avenae* burden than controls.

RNA interference (RNAi) is a method of gene silencing observed in a wide range of organisms. This method of gene silencing has become a useful tool for biologists to study biological processes and has been developed into a novel control strategy for engineering plants with nematode resistance. First identified in plants [154] the mechanism of action was elucidated in the nematode model organism *C. elegans* [155]. RNAi involves the suppression of specific transcripts to minimum expression levels as a method of post-transcriptional gene silencing during developmental processes and is believed to be a response to double-stranded viral entry. RNAi is premised on the cell's ability to recognize and degrade double-stranded RNA (dsRNA). The dsRNA is processed into small interfering RNA (siRNA) by the enzyme Dicer, a ribosome III-like enzyme. Double-stranded siRNA is unwound into two single-stranded RNAs and one strand serves as a guide which associates with the RNA-induced silencing complex (RISC). This complex associate with the specific complementary mRNA expressed in the cell where the RNAse H enzyme Argonaute degrades the mRNA resulting in gene silencing. Since the discovery of RNA-interference, researchers have developed transgenic constructs that specifically target genes for functional characterizations. More recently, plants have been engineered to expresses double-stranded RNA that silence important genes in plant-parasitic nematodes [156, 157]. As nematodes feed on the plant cytoplasm, the uptake of the siRNA triggers the endogenous RNAi mechanism within the nematode, silencing the target gene involved in infection [158]. The RNAi approach was applied, using sequence fragments from *M. incognita* genes that encode for two heat-shock protein 90 (HSP90) and isocitrate lyase (ICL). Heterologous expression of RNAi constructs in tobacco plants correlated to a significant level of resistance against *M. incognita*. Delayed galling and decreased egg production was observed in plants expressing HSP90 dsRNA. The *16D10* effector gene encodes for a secretory peptide synthesized in the subventral esophageal glands of root-knot nematodes which plays an important role in giant cell formation cells [156]. *In planta* expression of 16D10 dsRNA in Arabidopsis conferred in resistance effective against the four major root-knot nematode species [156]. In transgenic lines of potato expressing a 16D10 RNAi construct (Mc16D10L), the number of *M. chitwoodi* egg masses and eggs was significantly decreased in comparison to empty vector controls [159]. *Mc16D10L* expression was reduced in eggs and juveniles developed on transgenic potato which suggest a stable heritability of the construct. Decreased egg production was also observed in transgenic grape lines expressing *16D10L* [160].

http://dx.doi.org/10.5772/intechopen.68958

The use of site-specific DNA endonucleases including Zinc finger nucleases (ZFNs), [161] transcription activator-like effector nucleases (TALENs) [162] and now clustered regularly interspaced short palindromic repeats (CRISPR)/Cas9 [163] have equipped researchers with the ability to specifically inactivate genes and target genetic regions for homologous recombination of input DNA. In general, double-stranded breaks introduced by nucleases activates DNA repair mechanisms which generate mutations in the target sequence conferring a loss of expression i.e., gene editing. Homologous recombination of exogenously supplied sequences can result in genetic modifications (knock-ins). CRISPR technology has important advantages over TALENS and ZFNs including; ease of use [164] target site selection [165] and overall efficiency, although off-target effects remains an important issue of concern [166]. CRISPR/Cas9 system may be used to alter the expression of resistance genes for constitutive expression against plant-parasitic nematodes. For example, point mutations in the *snc1* (suppressor of npr1-1, constitutive 1) locus in *Arabidopsis* plants resulted in constitutive expression of pathogenesis-related proteins and enhanced disease resistance against two plant pathogens [167]. The mutation was mapped to a single nucleotide change in 120-kb region on chromosome 4 which contains a cluster of resistance genes. In a recent sweetpotato study, putative disease resistance gene *DRL23* showed elevated expression in resistant sweetpotato genotypes when compared to susceptible plants at days 14 and 46 post-inoculation with *Meloidogyne incognita* inoculum [168]. To identify any polymorphisms in amino sequences between *DRL23* from resistant and susceptible cultivars, protein alignments using the NCBI BLAST (Basic Local Alignment Search Tool) was performed. Interestingly, variations in amino acid sequences occurred between resistant (positions 187–231) and susceptible (positions 57–102) which corresponded to the NBS domain. Mutations in the NB-ARC domain often abolish R-protein function, indicative of the functional relevance of this domain [169]. Precise targeting by CRISPR may be useful in restoring gene function by sequence replacement in defense-related genes thereby enhancing resistance to nematode infection.

Acknowledgements

The authors would like to acknowledge the IBREED program under USDA-NIFA Grant #2014-38821-22448 and the Tuskegee University George Washington Carver Agricultural Experiment Station.

Author details

Gregory C. Bernard*, Marceline Egnin and Conrad Bonsi

Address all correspondence to: gbernard4673@mytu.tuskegee.edu

Tuskegee University, Tuskegee, Alabama, United States

References

[1] Hugot J, Baujard P, Morand S. Biodiversity in helminths and nematodes as a field of study: An overview. Nematology. 2001;**3**:199-208. DOI: 10.1163/156854101750413270

[2] Page A, Stepek G, Winter A, Pertab D. Enzymology of the nematode cuticle: A potential drug target? International Journal for Parasitology: Drugs and Drug Resistance. 2014;**4**:133-141. DOI: 10.1016/j.ijpddr.2014.05.003

[3] Kiontke K, Fitch D. Nematodes. Current Biology. 2013;**23**:862-864. DOI: http://dx.doi.org/10.1016/j.cub.2013.08.009

[4] Maier T, Hewezi T, Peng J, Baum TJ. Isolation of whole esophageal gland cells from plant-parasitic nematodes for transcriptome analyses and effector identification. Molecular Plant-Microbe Interactions. 2013;**26**:31-35. DOI: 10.1094/MPMI-05-12-0121-FI

[5] Poinar GO. 1983. The Natural History of Nematodes. Prentice Hall, Englewood Cliffs, NJ

[6] Noel GR. History, distribution, and economics. In: Riggs R, Wrather JA, editors. Biology and Management of the Soybean Cyst Nematode. American Phytopathological Society;1992. pp. 1-13

[7] Needham T. A Letter from Mr. Turbevil Needham, to the President; Concerning Certain Chalky Tubulous Concretions, Called Malm: With Some Microscopical Observations on the Farina of the Red Lily, and of Worms Discovered in Smutty Corn. Philosophical Transactions of the Royal Society of London. 1742;**42**:462-471 DOI:10.1098/rstl.1742.0101

[8] Berkeley M. Vibrio forming cysts on the roots of cucumbers. Gardeners' Chronicle. 1855; **7**:220

[9] Quentin M, Abad P, Favery B. Plant parasitic nematode effectors target host defense and nuclear functions to establish feeding cells. Frontiers in Plant Science. 2013;**4**:1-7. DOI: 10.3389/fpls.2013.00053

[10] Davis EL, Hussey RS, Mitchum MG and Baum TJ. Parasitism proteins in nematode-plant interactions. Current Opinion in Plant Biology. 2008;**11**:360-366. DOI: 10.1016/j.pbi.2008.04.003

[11] Abad P, Gouzy J, Aury J, Castagnone-Sereno P, Danchi EGJ, Deleury E, Perfus-Barbeoch L, Anthouard V, Artiguenave F, Blok VC, Caillaud MC, Coutinho PM, Dasilva C, De Luca F, Deau F, Esquibet M, Flutre T, Goldstone JV, Hamamouch N, Hewezi T, Jaillon O, Jubin C, Leonetti P, Magliano M, Maier TR, Markov GV, McVeigh P, Pesole G, Poulain J, Robinson-Rechavi M, Sallet E, Segurens B, Steinbach D, Tytgat T, Ugarte E, van Ghelder C, Veronico P, Baum TJ, Blaxter M, Bleve-Zacheo T, Davis EL, Ewbank JJ, Favery B, Grenier E, Henrissat B, Jones JT, Laudet V, Maule AG, Quesneville H, Rosso MN, Schiex T, Smant G, Weissenbach J, Wincker P. Genome sequence of the metazoan plant-parasitic nematode *Meloidogyne incognita*. Nature Biotechnology. 2008;**26**:909-915. DOI: 10.1038/nbt.1482

[12] Smant G, Stokkermans J, Yan Y, de Boer JM, Baum TJ, Wang X, Hussey R, Gommers F, Henrissat B, Davis E, Helder J, Schots A, Bakker J. Endogenous cellulases in animals: Isolation of β-1,4-endoglucanase genes from two species of plant-parasitic cyst nematodes. PNAS. 1998;**95**:4906-4911

[13] Yan Y, Smant G, Stokkermans J, Qin L, Helder J, Baum T, Schots A, Davis E. Genomic organization of four beta-1,4-endoglucanase genes in plant-parasitic cyst nematodes and its evolutionary implications. Gene. 1998;**220**:61-70

[14] Jones J, Furlanetto C, Kikuchi T. Horizontal gene transfer from bacteria and fungi as a driving force in the evolution of plant parasitism in nematodes. Nematology. 2005;**7**:642-646. DOI: 10.1163/156854105775142919

[15] Rybarczyk-Mydłowska K, Maboreke H, van Megen H, van den Elsen S, Mooyman P, Smant G, Bakker J, Helder J. Rather than by direct acquisition via lateral gene transfer, GHF5 cellulases were passed on from early Pratylenchidae to root-knot and cyst nematodes. BMC Evolutionary Biology. 2012;**12**:221. DOI: 10.1186/1471-2148-12-221

[16] Kikuchi T, Jones J, Aikawa T, Kosaka H, Ogura N. A family of glycosyl hydrolase family 45 cellulases from the pine wood nematode *Bursaphelenchus xylophilus*. FEBS Letters. 2004;**572**:201-205. DOI: 10.1016/j.febslet.2004.07.039

[17] Palomares-Rius J, Hirooka Y, Tsa I, Masuya H, Hino A, Kanzaki N, Jones J, Kikuchi T. Distribution and evolution of glycoside hydrolase family 45 cellulases in nematodes and fungi. BMC Evolutionary Biology. 2014;**14**: 69. DOI: 10.1186/1471-2148-14-69

[18] Villate L, Fievet V, Hanse B, Delemarre F, Plantard O, Esmenjaud D, van Helden M. Spatial distribution of the dagger nematode Xiphinema index and its associated Grapevine fanleaf virus in French vineyard. Phytopathology. 2008;**98**:942-948. DOI: 10.1094/PHYTO-98-8-0942

[19] Williamson V, Hussey R. Nematode pathogenesis and resistance in plants. The Plant Cell. 1996;**8**:1735-1745. DOI: 10.1105/tpc.8.10.1735

[20] Decraemer W, Hunt D. Structure and classification. In: Perry R, Moens M, editors. Plant Nematology. Oxfordshire: CAB International;2006. pp. 3-32. DOI: 10.1079/9781845930561.0000

[21] Nicol J, Turner D, Coyne L, den Nijs L, Hockland S, Maafi Z. Current nematode threats to world agriculture. In: Jones J, Gheysen G, Fenoll C, editors. Genomics and Molecular Genetics of Plant-Nematode Interactions. Berlin:Springer Science Business Media; 2011. pp. 21-43. DOI 10.1007/978-94-007-0434-3_2

[22] Sasser J, Freckman D. A world perspective on nematology: The role of the society. In: Veech J, Dickson D, editors. Vistas on Nematology; Society of Nematologists, Inc.: Hyattsville, MD .pp.7-14

[23] Koenning S, Overstreet C, Noling J, Donald P, Becker J, Fortnum B. Survey of crop losses in response to phytoparasitic nematodes in the United States for 1994. Journal of Nematology. 1999;**31**(4S): 587-618

[24] FAO. Cereal Supply and Demand Brief [Internet]. 2017. Available from: http://www.fao.org/worldfoodsituation/csdb/en/ [Accessed: 10-03-2017]

[25] Smiley R, Guiping Y. Cereal cyst nematodes. Biology and management in Pacific Northwest wheat, barley, and oat crops. A Pacific Northwest Extension Publication Oregon State University [Internet] 2010. Available from: http://ir.library.oregonstate.edu/xmlui/bitstream/handle/1957/18917/pnw620.pdf [Accessed: 15-03-2017]

[26] Bonfil D, Dolgin B, Mufradi I, Asido S. Bioassay to forecast cereal cyst nematode damage to wheat in fields. Precision Agriculture. 2004;**5**: 329-344. DOI: 10.1023/B:PRAG.0000040804.97462.02

[27] Nicol J, Elekçioğlu H, Bolat N, Rivoal R. The global importance of the cereal cyst nematode (*Heterodera* spp.) on wheat and international approaches to its control. Communications in Agricultural and Applied Biological Sciences. 2004;**72**: 677-686

[28] Lasserre, F, Rivoal, R, Cook, R. Interactions between Heterodera avenae and Pratylenchus neglectus on wheat. Journal of Nematology. 1994;**26**:336-344

[29] Riley T, Reardon T. Isolation and characterization of *Clavibacter tritici* associated with *Anguina tritici* in wheat from Western Australia. Plant Pathology. 1995;**44**: 805-810. DOI: 10.1111/j.1365-3059.1995.tb02739.x

[30] Childs, Nathan. 2017. U.S. 2016/17 Export Forecast Lowered 2.0 Million Cwt to 110.0 Million cwt. USDA-ERS Situation and Outlook. RCS-17B https://www.ers.usda.gov/webdocs/publications/rcs17b/rcs-17b.pdf?v=42787

[31] Trudgill D, Blok V. Apomictic, polyphagous root-knot nematodes: exceptionally successful and damaging biotrophic root pathogens. Annual Review of Phytopathology. 2001;**39**:53-77. doi: 10.1146/annurev.phyto.39.1.53

[32] Soriano I, Prot J, Matias D. Expression of tolerance for Meloidogyne graminicola in rice cultivars as affected by soil type and flooding. Journal of Nematology. 2000;**32**:309-317

[33] Pokharel R, Abawi G, Zhang N, Duxbury J, Smart, C. Characterization of isolates of *Meloidogyne* from rice-wheat production fields in Nepal. Journal of Nematology. 2007;**39**: 221-230

[34] Kyndt T, Fernandez D, Gheysen G. Plant-parasitic nematode infections in rice: Molecular and cellular insights. Annual Review of Phytopathology. 2014;**52**:135-153. DOI: 10.1146/annurev-phyto-102313-050111

[35] Bridge J Plowright R, Peng D. Nematode parasites of rice. In: Luc M, Sikora R, Bridge J, editors. Plant Parasitic Nematodes in Subtropical and Tropical Agriculture. 2nd ed. Egham:CABI Bioscience; 2005. pp. 87-130. DOI: 10.1079/9780851997278.0000

[36] Norton D. Maize nematode problems. Plant Disease. 1983;**67**:253-256

[37] Norton D, Hoffmann J. Longidorus breviannulatus n. sp. (Nematoda: Longidoridae) associated with stunted corn in Iowa. Journal of Nematology. 1975;**7**:168-171

[38] FAOSTAT. World production of potato. [Internet]. 2015. Available from http://www.nationalpotatocouncil.org/files/1114/4223/8719/Pg._78_World_Potato_Production.pdf [Accessed: 20-03-2017]

[39] Turner S, Evans K. The origins, global distribution and biology of potato cyst nematodes (*Globodera rostochiensis* (Woll.) and *G. pallida* Stone). In: Marks R, Brodie B. editors. Potato Cyst Nematodes: Biology, Distribution, and Control. Cambridge: University Press; 1998. pp. 7-26

[40] Jones L, Koehler A, Trnka M, Balek J, Challinor A, Atkinson H, Urwin P. Climate change is predicted to alter the current pest status of Globodera pallida and G. rostochiensis in the UK. Global Change Biology. DOI: 10.1111/gcb.13676

[41] Santo G, O'Bannon J, Finley A, Golden A. Occurrence and host range of a new root-knot nematode (*Meloidogyne chitwoodi*) in the Pacific Northwest. Plant Disease. 1980;**64**:951-952. DOI: 10.1094/PD-64-951

[42] Xu Z, Zhao Y, Yang D, Sun H, Zhang C, Xie Y. Attractant and repellent effects of sweet potato root exudates on the potato rot nematode, *Ditylenchus destructor*. Nematology. 2015;**17**:117-124. DOI: 10.1163/15685411-00002856

[43] Zhang S, Zhang S, Wang H, Chen Y. Characteristics of sweetpotato stem nematode in China. Acta Phytopathologica Sinica. 2006;**36**:22-27

[44] CIP International Potato Center. Sweetpotato Facts and Figures. 2014. Available from: http://cipotato.org/sweetpotato/facts-2/. [Accessed: 20-03-2017]

[45] Bonsi C, Phills B. Reaction of twelve sweetpotato cultivars and breeding lines to root-knot species with three experimental methods. HortScience. 1979;**14**:539-541

[46] Cervantes-Flores J, Yencho G, Davis E. Detection of quantitative trait loci and inheritance of root-knot nematode resistance in sweetpotato. HortScience. 2008;**133**:841-851

[47] Jones J, Haegeman A, Danchin E, Gaur H, Helder J, Jones M, Kikuchi T, Manzanilla-Lopez R, Palomares-Rius J, Wesemael W, Perry R. Top 10 plant-parasitic nematodes in molecular plant pathology. Molecular Plant Pathology.. 2013;**14**:946-961. DOI: 10.1111/mpp.12057

[48] Postnikova O, Hult M, Shao J, Skantar A, Nemchinov L. Transcriptome analysis of resistant and susceptible alfalfa cultivars infected with root-knot nematode Meloidogyne incognita. PloS One. 2015;**10**:e0118269. DOI: 10.1371/journal.pone.0118269

[49] Davis E, Hussey R, Baum T, Bakker J, Schots A, Rosso M, Abad P. Nematode parasitism genes. Annual Review of Phytopathology. 2000;**38**:365-396. DOI: 10.1146/annurev.phyto.38.1.365

[50] Caillaud M, Dubreuil G, Quentin M, Perfus-Barbeoch L, Lecomte P, de Almeida Engler J, Abad P, Rosso M, Favery B. Root-knot nematodes manipulate plant cell functions during a compatible interaction. Journal of Plant Physiology. 2008;**165**:104-113. DOI: 10.1016/j.jplph.2007.05.007

[51] Hewezi T, Baum T. Manipulation of plant cells by cyst and root-knot nematode effectors. Molecular Plant-Microbe Interactions. 2013;**26**:9-16. DOI: 10.1094/MPMI-05-12-0106-FI

[52] Gheysen G, Fenoll C. Gene expression in nematode feeding sites. Annual Review of Phytopathology. 2002;**40**:191-219. Epub 2002 Feb 20 DOI:10.1146/annurev.phyto.40.121201.093719

[53] Wrather A, Mitchum M. Soybean cyst nematodes: Diagnosis and Management. [Internet] 2010. Available from: http://extension.missouri.edu/p/g4450 [Accessed: 23-03-2017]

[54] PM 7/40 (3) *Globodera rostochiensis* and *Globodera pallida*. Bulletin OEPP/EPPO Bulletin. 2013:43. DOI: 10.1111/epp.12025

[55] Abawi G, Mai W. Effects of initial population densities of *Heterodera schachtii* on yield of cabbage and table beets in New York State. Phytopathology. 1980;**70**(6):481-485

[56] Muller J. The economic importance of *Heterodera schachtii* in Europe. Helminthologia. 1999; **36**(3):205-213

[57] Davis E, MacGuidwin A. Lesion nematode disease. The Plant Health Instructor. [Internet]. 2000. Available from: http://www.apsnet.org/edcenter/intropp/lessons/Nematodes/Pages/LesionNematode.aspx [Accessed: 23-03-2017]. DOI: 10.1094/PHI-I-2000-1030-02

[58] Smiley R. Root-lesion nematodes: Biology and management in Pacific Northwest wheat cropping systems. [Internet]. 2015. Available from: https://catalog.extension.oregonstate.edu/sites/catalog/files/project/pdf/pnw617_1.pdf. [Accessed: 23-03-2017]

[59] Jones M, Fosu-Nyarko J. Molecular biology of root lesion nematodes (Pratylenchus spp.) and their interaction with host plants. Annals of Applied Biology. 2014;**164**:163-181. DOI: 10.1111/aab.12105

[60] Kim D, Chun J, Lee KY. *Pratylenchus kumamotoensis* and *P. pseudocoffeae* (Nematoda, Pratylenchidae) newly recorded in Korea. Zookeys. 2016;**600**:1-5. DOI: 10.3897/zookeys.600.8508

[61] Smith I, Charles L, editors. Distribution Maps of Quarantine Pests for Europe. Wallingford: CABI International; 1998. pp. 1-78

[62] Sarah J, Gowen S, De Waele D, Tessera M, Quimio A. Nematode pathogens. In: Jones D, editors. Diseases of Banana, Abacá and Ensete. Wallingford: CABI Publishing; 1999. pp. 295-303

[63] Li Y, Wang K, Xie H, Wang Y, Wang D, Xu C, Huang X, Wang D. Nematode calreticulin, RsCRT is a key effector in reproduction and pathogenicity of *Radopholus similis*. PloS One. 2015;**10**:1-20. DOI: 10.1371/journal.pone.0129351.

[64] Hölscher D, Dhakshinamoorthy S, Alexandrov T, Becker M, Bretschneider T, Buerkert A, … Swennen R. Phenalenone-type phytoalexins mediate resistance of banana plants (*Musa spp.*) to the burrowing nematode *Radopholus similis*. PNAS. 2014;**11**:105-110. DOI: 10.1073/pnas.1314168110

[65] Gleason C, Polzin F, Habash S, Zhang L, Utermark J, Grundler F, Elashry A. Identification of two *Meloidogyne hapla* genes and an investigation of their roles in plant-nematode interaction. MPMI. 2017;**30**:101-112. DOI: http://dx.doi.org/10.1094/MPMI-06-16-0107-R

[66] Bashline L, Lei L, Li S, Gu Y. Cell wall, cytoskeleton, and cell expansion in higher plants. Molecular Plant. 2014;**7**:586-600. DOI: 10.1093/mp/ssu018

[67] Fudali S, Sobczak M, Janakowski S, Griesser M, Grundler FM, Golinowski W. Expansins are among plant cell wall modifying agents specifically expressed during development of nematode-induced syncytia. Plant Signaling & Behavior. 2008;**3**:969-971. DOI: 10.4161/psb.6169

[68] Liu J, Peng H, Cui J, Huang W, Kong L, Clark J, Jian H, Wang G, Peng D. Molecular characterization of a novel effector expansin-like protein from *Heterodera avenae* that induces cell death in *Nicotiana benthamiana*. Scientific Reports. 2016;**6**:35677. DOI: 10.1038/srep35677

[69] Zheng M, Long H, Zhao Y, Lin L, Xu D, Zhang H, Liu F, Deng G, Pan Z, Yu M. RNA-Seq based identification of candidate parasitism genes of cereal cyst nematode (*Heterodera avenae*) during incompatible infection to *Aegilops variabilis*. PloS One. 2015;**10**:e0141095. DOI: http://doi.org/10.1371/journal.pone.0141095

[70] Guan T, Shen J, Fa Y, Su Y, Wang X, Li H. Resistance-breaking population of *Meloidogyne incognita* utilizes plant peroxidase to scavenge reactive oxygen species, thereby promoting parasitism on tomato carrying Mi-1 gene. Biochemical and Biophysical Research Communications 2017;**482**:1-7. DOI: 10.1016/j.bbrc.2016.11.040

[71] Lacomme C, Santa Cruz S. Bax-induced cell death in tobacco is similar to the hypersensitive response. PNAS. 1999;**96**:7956-7961. DOI: 10.1073/pnas.96.14.7956

[72] Li X, Yang D, Niu J, Zhao J, Jian H. De novo analysis of the transcriptome of *Meloidogyne enterolobii* to uncover potential target genes for biological control. International Journal of Molecular Sciences. 2016;**17**:1442. DOI: 10.3390/ijms17091442

[73] Postma W, Slootweg E, Rehman S, Finkers-Tomczak A, Tytgat T, Van Gelderen K, Lozano-Torress J, Roosien J, Pomp R, van Schaik C, Bakker J, Goverse A, Smant G. The effector SPRYSEC-19 of *Globodera rostochiensis* suppresses CC-NB-LRR-mediated disease resistance in plants. Plant Physiology. 2012;**160**:944-954. DOI: 10.1104/pp.112.200188

[74] Ali S, Magne M, Chen S, Obradovic N, Jamshaid L, Wang X, Belair G, Moffett P. Analysis of Globodera rostochiensis effectors reveals conserved functions of SPRYSEC proteins in suppressing and eliciting plant immune responses. Frontiers in Plant Science. 2015;**6**:623. DOI: 10.3389/fpls.2015.00623

[75] Milligan S, Bodeau J, Yaghoobi J, Kaloshian I, Zabel P, Williamson V. The root-knot nematode resistance gene Mi from tomato is a member of the leucne zipper, nucleotide binding, leucine-rich repeat family of plant genes. Plant Cell. 1998;**10**:1307-1319

[76] Cai D, Kleine M, Kifle S, Harloff H, Sandal N, Marcker K, Klein-Lankhorst R, Salentijn E, Lange W, Stiekema W, Wyss U, Grundler F, Jung C. Positional cloning of a gene for nematode resistance in sugar beet. Science. 1997;**275**:832-834

[77] Van der Vossen E, van der Voort J, Kanyuka K, Bendahmane A, Sandbrink H, Baulcombe D, Bakker J, Stiekema W, Klein-Lankhorst R. Homologues of a single resistance-gene

cluster in potato confer resistance to distinct pathogens: A virus and a nematode. The Plant Journal. 2000;**23**:567-576. DOI: 10.1046/j.1365-313x.2000.00814.x

[78] Paal J, Henselewski H, Muth J, Meksem K, Menendez C, Salamini F, Ballvora A, Gebhardt C. Molecular cloning of the potato Gro1-4 gene conferring resistance to pathotype Ro1 of the root cyst nematode *Globodera rostochiensis*, based on a candidate gene approach. The Plant Journal. 2004;**38**:285-287. DOI: 10.1111/j.1365-313X.2004.02047.x

[79] Smith P. Embryo culture of a tomato species hybrid. Proceedings of the American Society for Horticultural Sciences. 1944;**44**: 413-416

[80] Frazier W, Dennett R. Isolation of Lycopersicon esculentum type tomato lines essentially homozygous resistant to root-knot. Proceedings of the American Society for Horticultural Science. 1949;**54**:225-236

[81] Rossi M, Goggin F, Milligan S, Kaloshian I, Ullman D, Williamson V. The nematode resistance gene *Mi* of tomato confers resistance against the potato aphid. Proceedings of the National Academy of Sciences of the United States of America. 1998;**95**: 9750-9754

[82] Nombela G, Williamson V, Muniz M. The root-knot nematode resistance gene Mi-1.2 of tomato is responsible for resistance against the whitefly *Bemisia tabaci*. Molecular Plant-Microbe Interactions. 2003;**16**:645-649. DOI: 10.1094/MPMI.2003.16.7.645

[83] Martinez de Illarduya O, Nombela G, Hwang C, Williamson V, Muniz M, Kaloshian I. Rme1 is necessary for Mi-1 resistance and acts early in the resistance pathway. Molecular Plant-Microbe Interactions. 2004;**17**:55-61. DOI: 10.1094/MPMI.2004.17.1.55

[84] Ali A, Matthews W, Cavagnaro P, Iorizzo M, Roberts P, Simon P. Inheritance and mapping of Mj-2, a new source of root-knot nematode (*Meloidogyne javanica*) resistance in carrot. Journal of Heredity. 2014;**105**:288-291. DOI: 10.1093/jhered/est090

[85] Simon P, Matthews W, Roberts P. Evidence for simply inherited dominant resistance to *Meloidogyne javanica* in carrot. Theoretical and Applied Genetics. 2000;**100**:735-742. DOI:10.1007/s001220051346

[86] Duval H, Hoerter M, Polidori J, Confolent C, Masse M, Moretti A, Van Ghelder C, Esmenjaud D. High-resolution mapping of the RMia gene for resistance to root-knot nematodes in peach. Tree Genetics and Genomes. 2014;**10**:297-306. DOI: 10.1007/s11295-013-0683-z

[87] Claverie M, Dirlewanger E, Bosselut N, Van Ghelder C, Voisin R, Kleinhentz M, Lafargue B, Abad P, Rosso M, Chalhoub B, Esmenjaud D. The Ma gene for complete-spectrum resistance to Meloidogyne species in Prunus is a TNL with a huge repeated C-terminal post-LRR region. Plant Physiology. 2011;**156**:779-792. DOI: 10.1104/pp.111.176230

[88] Claverie M, Bosselut N, Lecouis A, Voisin R, Lafargue B, Poizat C, Kleinhentz M, Laigret F, Dirlewanger E, Esmenjaud D. Location of independent root-knot nematode resistance genes in plum and peach. Theoretical and Applied Genetics. 2004;**108**:765-773. DOI: 10.1007/s00122-003-1463-1

[89] Yang Y, Rosen B, Scoffield J, He G. Isolation and analysis of resistance gene homologues in sweetpotato. Plant Breeding. 2010;**129**:519-525 DOI: 10.1111/j.1439-0523.2009.01711.x

[90] Michelmore R, Paran I, Kesseli R. Identification of markers linked to disease-resistance genes by bulked segregant analysis: A rapid method to detect markers in specific genomic regions by using segregating populations. PNAS. 1991;**88**:9828-9832. DOI: 10.1073/pnas.88.21.9828

[91] Ukoskit K, Thompson P, Watson C. Identifying a randomly amplified polymorphic DNA (RAPD) marker linked to a gene for root-knot nematode resistance in sweetpotato. Journal of the American Society of Horticultural Science. 1997;**122**:818-821

[92] Mauricio R, Stahl E, Korves T, Tian D, Kreitman M, Bergelson J. Natural selection for polymorphism in the disease resistance gene Rps2 of *Arabidopsis thaliana*. Genetics. 2003;**163**:735-746

[93] Kawahara Y, Oono Y, Kanamori H, Matsumoto T, Itoh T, Minami E. Simultaneous RNA-Seq analysis of a mixed transcriptome of rice and blast fungus interaction. PLoS One. 2012;**7**:e49423

[94] Yang F, Li W, Jorgensen H. Transcriptional reprogramming of wheat and the hemibiotrophic pathogen Septoria tritici during two phases of the compatible interaction. PLoS One. 2013;**8**:e81606. DOI: 10.1371/journal.pone.0081606

[95] Oliveira J, Andrade N, Martins-Miranda A, Soares A, Gondim D, Araujo-Filho J, Freire-Filho F, Vasconcelos I. Differential expression of antioxidant enzymes and PR-proteins in compatible and incompatible interactions of cowpea (*Vigna unguiculate*) and the root-knot nematode *Meloidogyne incognita*. Plant Physiology and Biochemistry. 2012;**51**:145-152. DOI: 10.1016/j.plaphy.2011.10.008

[96] Li R, Rashotte A, Singh N, Lawrence K, Weaver D, Locy R. Transcriptome analysis of cotton (*Gossypium hirsutum* L.) genotypes that are susceptible, resistant and hypersensitive to reniform nematode (*Rotylenchulus reniformis*). PloS One. 2015;**10**:1-27. DOI: 10.1371/journal.pone.014326

[97] Petitot A, Dereeper A, Agbessi M, Da Silva C, Guy J, Ardisson M, Fernandez D. Dual RNA-seq reveals Meloidogyne graminicola transcriptome and candidate effectors during the interaction with rice plants. Molecular Plant Pathology. 2016;**17**:860-874. DOI: 10.1111/mpp.12334

[98] Wan J, Vuong T, Jiao Y, Joshi T, Zhang H, Xu D, Nguyen H. Whole-genome gene expression profiling revealed genes and pathways potentially involved in regulating interactions of soybean with cyst nematode (*Heterodera glycines* Ichinohe). BMC Genomics. 2015;**16**:1-14. DOI: 10.1186.s12864-015-1316-8

[99] Xing X, Li X, Zhang M, Wang Y, Liu B, Xi Q, Zhao D, Wu Y, and Yang T. Transcriptome analysis of resistant and susceptible tobacco (*Nicotiana tabacum*) in response to root-

knot nematode *Meloidogyne incognita* infection. Biochemical and Biophysical Research Communications. 2017: **482**:1114-1121. DOI: 10.1016/j.bbrc.2016.11.167

[100] Dangl J, Jones J. Plant pathogens and integrated defence responses to infection. Nature. 2001;**411**:826-833. DOI: 10.1038/35081161

[101] Melillo M, Leonetti P, Bongiovanni M, Castagnone-Sereno P, Bleve-Zacheo T. Modulation of reactive oxygen species activities and H_2O_2 accumulation during compatible and incompatible tomato-root-knot nematode interactions. New Phytologist. 2006;**170**:501-512. DOI: 10.1111/j.1469-8137.2006.01724

[102] Kawano T. Roles of the reactive oxygen species-generating peroxidase reactions in plant defense and growth induction. Plant Cell Reports. 2003;**21**:829-837.DOI:10.1007/s00299-003-0591-z

[103] Simonetti E, Veronico P, Melillo M, Delibes A, Andres M, López-Braña I. Analysis of class III peroxidase genes expressed in roots of resistant and susceptible wheat lines infected by *Heterodera avenae*. MPMI. 2009;**22**:1081-1092. DOI:10.1094/MPMI -22-9-1081

[104] Graham M, Graham T. Rapid accumulation of anionic peroxidases and phenolic polymers in soybean cotyledon tissues following treatment with Phytophtora megasperma f. sp. Glycinea wall glucan. Plant Physiology. 1991;**94**:1445-1455. DOI:0032-0889/91/97/1445/11

[105] Zacheo G, Orlando C, Bleve-Zacheo T. Characterization of anionic peroxidases in tomato isolines infected by *Meloidogyne incognita*. Journal of Nematology. 1993;**25**:249-256

[106] van Loon L, van Strien E. The families of pathogenesis-related proteins, their activities, and comparative analysis of PR-1 type proteins. Physiological and Molecular Plant Pathology. 1999;**55**:85-97. http://dx.doi.org/10.1006/pmpp.1999.0213

[107] Van Loon L, Van Kammen A. Polyacrylamide disc electrophoresis of the soluble leaf proteins from Nicotiana tabaum var. 'Samsun' and 'Samsun NN'. II, Changes in protein constitution after in infection with TMV. Virology. 1970;**40**:199-201

[108] Gianinazzi S, Martin C, Vallee J. Hypersensibilite aux virus, temperature et proteins solubles chez le Nicotiana xanthi n.c. Apparition de nouvelles macromolecules lors de la repression de la synthese virale. Comptes Rendus de l'Académie des Sciences. 1970;**270**:2383-2386

[109] Molinari S, Fanelli E, Leonetti P. Expression of tomato salicylic acid (SA)-responsive pathogenesis-related genes in Mi-1-mediated and SA-induced resistance to root-knot nematodes. Molecular Plant Pathology. 2014;**152**:55-64. DOI: 10.1111/mpp.12085

[110] Uehara T, Sugiyama S, Matsuura H, Arie T, Masuta C. Resistant and susceptible responses in tomato to cyst nematode are differentially regulated by salicylic acid. Plant & Cell Physiology. 2010;**51**:1524-1536. DOI: 10.1093/pcp/pcq109

[111] Hi J, Kyndt T, He W, Vanholme B, Gheysen G. B-aminobutyric acid-induced resistance against root-knot nematodes in rice is based on increased basal defense. MPMI. 2015;**28**:519-533. DOI: 10.1094/MPMI-09-14-0260-R

[112] Amjad Ali M, Abbas A, Kreil D, Bohlmann H. Overexpression of the transcription factor RAP2.6 leads to enhanced callose deposition in syncytia and enhanced resistance against the beet cyst nematode *Heterodera schachtii* in *Arabidopsis* roots. BMC Plant Biology. 2013;**13**:1-17. DOI: 10.1186/1471-2229-13-47

[113] Rushton P, Torres J, Parniske M, Wernert P, Halhlbrock K, Somssich I. Interaction of elicitor-induced DNA-binding proteins with elicitor response elements in the promoters of parsley PR1 genes. EMBO Journal. 1996;**15**:5690-5700

[114] Atamian H, Eulgem T, Kaloshian I. SIWRKY70 is required for Mi-1 mediated resistance to aphids and nematodes in tomato. Planta 2012;**235**:299-309. DOI: 10.1007/s00425-011-1509-6

[115] Bhattarai K, Atamian H, Kaloshian I, Eulgem T. WRKY72-type transcription factors contribute to basal immunity in tomato and Arabidopsis as well as gene-for-gene resistance mediated by the tomato R gene Mi-1. The Plant Journal. 2010;**63**:229-240. DOI: 10.1111/j.1365-313X.2010.04232

[116] Grunewald W, Karimi M, Wieczorek K, Van de Cappelle E, Wischnitzki E, Grundler F, Inze D, Beeckman T, Gheysen G. A role for AtWRKY23 in feeding site establishment of plant-parasitic nematodes. Plant Physiology. 2008;**146**:358-368. DOI: 10.1104/pp.108.119131

[117] Amjad Ali M, Wieczorek K, Kreil D, Bohlmann H. The beet cyst nematode *Heterodera schachtii* modulates the expression of WRKY transcription factors in syncytia to favour its development in Arabidopsis roots. PLoS One. 2014;**9**:e102360. DOI: 10.1371/journal.pone.0102360

[118] Michalak M, Corbett E, Mesaeli N, Nakamura K, Opas M. Calreticulin: one protein, one gene, many functions. Biochemical Journal. 1999;**344**:281-291

[119] Saijo Y, Tintor N, Lu X, Rauf P, Pajerowska-Mukhtar K, Haweker H, Dong X, Robatzek S, Schulze-Lefert P. Receptor quality control in the endoplasmic reticulum for plant innate immunity. EMBO Journal. 2009;**28**:3439-3449. DOI: 10.1038/emboj.2009.263

[120] Christensen A, Svensson K, Thelin L, Zhang W, Tintor N, Prins D, Funke N, Michalak M, Schulze-Lefert P, Saijo Y, Sommarin M, Widell S, Persson S. Higher plant calreticulins have acquired specialized functions in Arabidopsis. PLoS One. 2010;**5**:e11342. DOI: 10.1371/journal.pone.0011342

[121] Jaouannet M, Magliano M, Arguel M, Gourgues M, Evangelisti E, Abad P, Rosso M. The root-knot nematode calreticulin Mi-CRT is a key effector in plant defense suppression. Molecular Plant-Microbe Interactions. 2013;**26**:97-105. DOI: 10.1094/MPMI-05-12-0130-R

[122] Laskowski M, Kato I. Protein inhibitors of proteinases. Annual Review of Biochemistry. 1980;**49**:593-626. DOI: 10.1146/annurev.bi.49.070180.003113

[123] Mickel C, Standish J. Susceptibility of processed soy flour and soy grits in storage to attack by *Tribolium castaneum*. University of Minnesota Agricultural Experimental Station Technical Bulletin. 1947, **178**: 1-20

[124] Hepher, A., Atkinson HJ. 1992. Nematode control with proteinase inhibitors. European Patent Application Number 92301890.7, Publication Number 0 502 730 A1

[125] Urwin P, McPherson M, Atkinson H. Enhanced transgenic plant resistance to nematodes by dual proteinase inhibitor constructs. Planta. 1998;**204**:472-479. DOI: 10.1007/s004250050281

[126] Chan Y, Yang A, Chen J, Yeh K, Chan M. Heterologous expression of taro cystatin protects transgenic tomato against *Meloidogyne incognita* infection by means of interfering sex determination and supressing gall formation. Plant Cell Reports. 2010;**29**:231-238. DOI: 10.1007/s00299-009-0815-y

[127] Senthilkumar R, Yeh K. Multiple biological functions of sporamin related to stress tolerance in sweetpotato (Ipomoea batatas Lam). Biotechnology Advances. 2012;**30**:1309-1317. DOI: 10.1016/j.biotechadv.2012.01.022

[128] Yeh K, Chen J, Lin M, Chen Y, Lin C. Functional activity of sporamin from sweetpotato (Ipomoea batatas Lam.): A tuber storage protein with trypsin inhibitory activity. Plant Molecular Biology. 1997;**33**:565-570

[129] Cai D, Thurau T, Tian Y, Lange T, Yeh K, Jung C. Sporamin-mediated resistance to beet cyst nematodes (Heterodera schachtii Schm.) is dependent on trypsin inhibitory activity in sugar beet (Beta vulgaris L.) hairy roots. Plant Molecular Biology. 2003;**51**:839-849. DOI: 10.1023/A:1023089017906

[130] Loake G, Grant M. Salicylic acid in plant defence-the players and protagonists. Current Opinion in Plant Biology. 2007;**10**:466-472. DOI: 10.1016/j.pbi.2007.08.008

[131] Liao Y, Tiam M, Zhang H, Li X, Wang Y, Xia X, Zhou J, Zhou Y, Yu J, Shi K, Klessig D. Salicylic acid binding of mitochondrial alpha-ketoglutarate dehydrogenase E2 affects mitochondrial oxidative phosphorylation and electron transport chain components and plays a role in basal defense against tobacco mosaic virus in tomato. New Phytologist. 2015;**205**:1296-1307. DOI: 10.1111/nph.13137

[132] Glazebrook J. Contrasting mechanisms of defense against biotrophic and necrotrophic pathogens. Annual Review of Phytopathology. 2005;**43**:205-227. DOI: 10.1146/annurev.phyto.43.040204.135923

[133] Nahar K, Kyndt T, De Vleesschauwer D, Hofte M, Gheysen G. The jasmonate pathway is a key player in systemically induced defense against root-knot nematodes in rice. Plant Physiology. 2011;**157**:305-316. DOI: 10.1104/pp.111.177576

[134] Vasyukova N, Zinovieva S, Udalova Z, Gerasimova N, Ozeretskovskaya O, Sonin M. Jasmonic acid and tomato resistance to the root-knot nematode *Meloidogyne incognita*. Doklady Biological Sciences. 2009;**428**:448-450. DOI: 10.1134/S0012496609050160

[135] Branch C, Hwang C, Navarre D, Williamson V. Salicylic acid is part of the Mi-1-mediated defense response to root-knot nematode in tomato. Molecular Plant-Microbe Interactions. 2004;**7**:351-356

[136] Sikora R, Fernandez E. Nematode parasites of vegetables. In: Luc M, Sikora R, Bridge J, editors. Plant parasitic nematodes in subtropical and tropical. Wallingford: CABI; 2005. pp. 319-392. DOI: dx.doi.org/10.1079/9780851997278.0000

[137] Osei K, Gowen S, Pembroke B, Brandenburg R, Jordan D. Potential of leguminous cover crops in management of a mixed population of root-knot nematodes (*Meloidogyne* spp.). Journal of Nematology. 2010;**42**:173-178

[138] Chen P, Tsay T. Effect of crop rotation on Meloidogyne spp. and Pratylenchus spp. populations in strawberry fields in Taiwan. Journal of Nematology. 2006;**38**:339-344

[139] Khan A, Sayed M,. Shaukat S, Handoo Z. Efficacy of four plant extracts on nematodes associated with papaya in Sindh, Pakistan. Nematologia Mediterranea 2008;**36**:93-98

[140] Okeniyi M, Afolami S, Fademi O, Oduwaye O. Effect of botanical extracts on root-knot nematode (*Meloidogyne incognita*) infection and growth of cashew (Anacardium occidentale) seedlings. Academia Journal of Biotechnology. 2013;**1**:81-86

[141] Bawa J, Mohammed I, Liadi S. Nematicidal effect of some plants extracts on root-knot nematodes (*Meloidogyne incognita*) of tomato (Lycopersicon esculentum). World Journal of Life Science and Medical Research. 2014;**3**:81-87

[142] Stirling G. Biological Control of Plant-parasitic Nematodes. Wallingford: CAB International; 1991. 282 p

[143] Meyer S. United States Department of Agriculture – Agricultural Research Service research programs on microbes for management of plant-parasitic nematodes. Pest Management Science. 2003;**59**:665-670

[144] Chen Z, Dickson D. Review of Pasteuria penetrans: Biology, ecology, and biological control potential. Journal of Nematology. 1998;**30**:313-340

[145] Kokalis-Burelle N. Pasteuria penetrans for control of *Meloidogyne incognita* on tomato and cucumber and M. arenaria on snapdragon. Journal of Nematology. 2015;**47**:207-213

[146] Weibelzahl-Fulton E, Dickson D, Whitty E. Suppression of *Meloidogyne incognita* and *M. javanica* by Pasteuria penetrans in field soil. Journal of Nematology. 1996;**28**:43-49

[147] Gao H, Qi G, Yin R, Zhang H, Li C, Zhao X. Bacillus cereus strain S2 shows high nematicidal activity against *Meloidogyne incognita* by producing sphingosine. Scientific Reports. 2016;**6**:28756. DOI: 10.1038/srep28756

[148] Xiong J, Zhou Q, Luo H, Xia L, Li L, Sun M, Yu Z. Systemic nematicidal activity and biocontrol efficacy of Bacillus firmus against the root-knot nematode *Meloidogyne incognita*.World Journal of Microbiology and Biotechnology. 2015;**31**:661-667. DOI: 10.1007/s11274-015-1820-7

[149] Atkins S, Hidalgo-Diaz L, Kalisz H, Mauchline T, Hirsch P, Kerry B. Development of a new management strategy for the control of root-knot nematodes (Meloidogyne spp) in organic vegetable production. Pest Management Science. 2003;**59**:183-189. DOI:10.1002/ps.603

[150] Gan Z, Yang J, Tao N, Liang L, Mi Q, Li J, Zhang K. Cloning of the gene Lecanicillium psalliotae chitinase Lpchi1 and identification of its potential role in the biocontrol of root-knot nematode *Meloidogyne incognita*. Applied Microbiology and Biotechnology. 2007;**76**:1309-1317. DOI:10.1007/s00253-007-1111-9

[151] Vishnudasan D, Tripathi M, Rao U, Khurana P. Assessment of nematode resistance in wheat transgenic plants expressing potato proteinase inhibitor (PIN2) gene. Transgenic Research. 2005;**14**:665-675. DOI:10.1007/s11248-005-5696-4

[152] Matthews B, Beard H, Brewer E, Kabir S, MacDonald M, Youssef R. Arabidopsis genes, AtNPR1, AtTGA2 and AtPR-5, confer partial resistance to soybean cyst nematode (*Heterodera glycines*) when overexpressed in transgenic soybean roots. BMC Plant Biology. 2014;**14**:1-19. DOI: 10.1186/1471-2229-14-96

[153] Lin J, Wang D, Chen X, Kollner T, Mazarei M, Guo H, Pantalone V, Arellii P, Stewart C, Chen F. An (E,E)-@-farnesene synthase gene of soybean has a role in defence against nematodes and is involved in synthesizing insect-induced volatiles. Plant Biotechnology Journal. 2017;**15**:510-519. DOI: 10.1111/pbi.12649

[154] Ecker J, Davis R. Inhibition of gene expression in plant cells by expression of antisense RNA. PNAS. 1986;**83**:5372-5376. DOI:10.1073/pnas.83.15.5372

[155] Fire A, SiQun X, Montgomery M, Kostas S, Driver S, Mello C. Potent and specific genetic inferference by double-stranded RNA in Caenorhabditis elegans. Nature. 1998;**391**:806-811. DOI: 10.1038/35888

[156] Huang G, Allen R, Davis E, Baum T, Hussey R. Engineering broad root-knot resistance in transgenic plants by RNAi silencing of a conserved and essential root-knot nematode parasitism gene. PNAS. 2006;**103**:14302-14306. DOI:10.1073/pnas.0604698103

[157] Yadav B, Veluthambi K, Subramaniam K. Host-generated double stranded RNA induces RNAi in plant-parasitic nematodes and protects the host from infection. Molecular & Biochemical Parasitology. 2006;**148**:219-222. DOI:10.1016/j.molbiopara.2006.03.013

[158] Lilley C, Davis L, Urwin P. RNA interference in plant parasitic nematodes: a summary of the current status. Parasitology. 2012;**139**:630-640. DOI: 10.1017/S0031182011002071

[159] Dinh P, Brown C, Elling A. RNA interference of effector gene Mc16D10L confers resistance against *Meloidogyne chitwoodi* in Arabidopsis and potato. Phytopathology. 2014;**104**:1098-1106. DOI: http://dx.doi.org/10.1094/PHYTO-03-14-0063-R

[160] Yang Y, Jittayasothorn Y, Chronis D, Wang X, Cousins P, Zhong G. Molecular characteristics and efficacy of 16D10 siRNAs in inhibiting root-knot nematode infection in transgenic grape hairy roots. PLoS One. 2013;**8**:e69463. DOI: 10.1371/journal.pone.0069463

[161] Bibikova M, Beumer K, Trautman JK, Carroll D. Enhancing gene targeting with designed zinc finger nucleases. Science. 2003;**300**:764. DOI:10.1126/science.1079512

[162] Forsyth A, Weeks T, Richael C, Duan H. Transcription activator-like effector nucleases (TALEN)-mediated targeted DNA insertion in potato plants. Frontiers in Plant Science. 2016;**7**:1572. DOI: 10.3389/fpls.2016.01572

[163] Redman M, King A, Watson C, King D. What is CRISPR/Cas9?. Archives of Disease in Childhood. Education and Practice Edition. 2016;**101**:213-215. DOI: 10.1136/archdischild-2016-310459

[164] Gupta R, Musunuru K. Expanding the genetic editing tool kit: ZFNs, TALENs, and CRISPR-Cas9. Journal of Clinical Investigation. 2014;**124**:4154-4161. DOI: 10.1172/JCI72992

[165] Mali P, Yang L, Esvelt K, Aach J, Guell M, DiCarlo J, Norville J, Church G. RNA-guided human genome engineering via Cas9. Science. 2013;**339**:823-826. DOI: 10.1126/science.1232033

[166] Fu Y, Foden J, Khayter C, Maeder M, Reyon D, Joung J, Sander J. High-frequency off-target mutagenesis induced by CRISPR-Cas nucleases in human cells. Nature Biotechnology. 2013;**31**:822-826. DOI: 10.1038/nbt.2623

[167] Zhang Y, Goritschnig S, Dong X, Li X. A Gain-of-Function Mutation in a Plant Disease Resistance Gene Leads to Constitutive Activation of Downstream Signal Transduction Pathways in suppressor of npr1-1, constitutive 1. The Plant Cell. 2003;**15**:2636-2646. DOI: http://doi.org/10.1105/tpc.015842

[168] Bernard G, Egnin M, Bonsi C, Mortley D, Witola W, Samuels S, Land C, Lawrence K. Efficient evaluation of physical and molecular plant immune responses to root-knot nematode infection in selected sweetpotato cultivars. In Vitro Cellular & Developmental Biology. 2016;**52**:437. DOI:10.1007/s11627-016-9771-8

[169] Dinesh-Kumar S, Tham W, Baker B. Structure-function analysis of the tobacco mosaic virus resistance gene N. PNAS. 2000;**97**:14789-14794. DOI: 10.1073/pnas.97.26.14789

Chapter 8

Harnessing Useful Rhizosphere Microorganisms for Nematode Control

Seloame Tatu Nyaku, Antoine Affokpon,
Agyemang Danquah and Francis Collison Brentu

Additional information is available at the end of the chapter

http://dx.doi.org/10.5772/intechopen.69164

Abstract

Nematodes are very diverse and parasitize various plants including vegetables, and their management is of concern. Biological control of nematodes provides an environmentally friendly management option and there are various micro-soil-borne organisms which can be considered for this purpose. The primary goal of this chapter is to provide a review on the progress made so far, in application of biological control agents in nematode management in vegetables, cereals, and root and tuber crops. This chapter will be divided into five (5) sections: (1) herbivore-induced plant volatiles, (2) root exudates and nematode control, (3) inhibitory metabolites in bacteria for nematode management, (4) fungi and symbiotic reprogramming in host cells, and (5) fungi antagonists of nematodes.

Keywords: arbuscular mycorrhizal fungi (AMF), biocontrol, volatile organic compounds (VOCs)

1. Introduction

Plant-parasitic nematodes (PPNs) represent serious threat to the world economy and are responsible for great losses in production systems worldwide [1]. In monetary terms, world agricultural economy losses are approximately $215.8 billion annually, because of 12.6% crop loss inflicted on top 20 life-sustaining crops by PPN based on 2010–2013 production figures and prices. These figures do not cover all crops throughout the world especially crops produced in the developing countries which will probably exceed these estimates if combined. Therefore, nematode management is a major constraint in food security efforts worldwide. However, PPNs are difficult to control compared to other pests because nematodes mostly inhabit the soil, and usually attack the underground parts of the plants [2]. Although chemical nematicides are effective, easy to apply, and show rapid effects, the growing dissatisfaction with chemical nematicides due to environmental and health issues has created redirections in the type and choice of applicable nematicides [3]. In view of these challenges posed by traditional nematicides, for the past 20 years the search for novel, environmentally friendly alternatives with which to manage PPN populations has therefore become increasingly important. The role of different beneficial microorganisms in the soil ranks high as environmentally friendly biological alternatives to synthetic nematicides [3].

Volatile compounds are emitted both by eukaryotes and by prokaryotes; these volatile organic compounds (VOCs) are lipophilic, with a molecular mass of about 300 Da or less, and a vapor pressure of 0.01 kPa. These chemicals evaporate easily and are produced through diffusion; however, other mechanisms (passive or active) for their emission and transmission exist [4]. Three chemical groups can be associated with the volatile compounds (terpenoids, phenylpropanoids, and fatty acid derivatives). Volatile compound penetration and movement in soils is greatly influenced by the mineral type, soil texture, and particle design [5]. The rhizosphere has within it various microorganisms because of its conducive environment; furthermore, about 20% of carbon can be released by roots [6]. Root exudates are made up of various chemical compounds, among these are amino acids and amides, organic acids, sugars, phenols, polysaccharides, secondary metabolites, and proteins [7]. Volatile metabolites effused in the soil could have an impact on the organism within the soil community. Mycorrhizal and non-mycorrhizal plants also release distinct root exudates which contain organic acids and sugars [8].

Plant-parasitic nematodes move toward their host and this phenomenon is important in agriculture [9]. Carbon dioxide is a root volatile with specific roles in luring plant-parasitic nematodes, for example, to their hosts *Meloidogyne incognita* [10], *Caenorhabditis elegans* [11], and *Ditylenchus dipsaci* [12]. In a previous study, a tracking system linked to a computer was implored to monitor the responses of second-stage juveniles of *M. incognita* exposed to carbon dioxide [10]. Results revealed a positive correlation among carbon dioxide concentration increase and nematode locomotion rate. Higher carbon dioxide concentrations (>10%) resulted in a reduction of nematode movement. In a second experiment, the movement of nematodes was monitored on a gradient, maintaining the carbon dioxide concentration constant. Thresholds were maintained either above or below 0.01% CO_2/cm. The migration rate under optimal CO_2concentrations was 0.7 cm/h. Plants secrete chemicals, for example, benzaldehyde, thymol, limonene, neral, geranial, and carvacrol which are needed for defense against other pathogens in the soil [13–18]. These chemicals may have within them nematicidal properties.

2. Herbivore-induced plant volatiles

Herbivore-induced plant volatiles (HIPVs) are generated after a herbivore feeds on its host roots and their roles to attract nematodes and other predators are still been explored [19–21]. Lima bean (*Phaseolus lunatus*) releases volatiles after the feeding activities of spider mites (*Tetranychus urticae*); this volatile attracts *Phytoseiulus persimilis* which is a predatory mite [22].

Among the compounds present in the oral secretions of herbivores are volicitin and fatty acid amides, which stimulate volatile release in plants [23, 24].

The roles herbivores play in relation to nematode parasitism on plants have been investigated [25, 26]. Signals released from plant roots, which are also parasitized by insects, influence the actions of entomopathogenic nematodes (EPNs) [27, 28]. Feeding mechanisms of herbivores stimulate the release of EPN-attracting volatiles, especially in annual grasses [29]. A hybrid root stock "*Swingle citrumelo*" lures EPNs (*Steinernema diaprepesi*) toward its roots after parasitism by larval *Diaprepes abbreviatus* root weevils; this is because of the production of subterranean volatiles (terpenoid) [30]. The citrus nematode *Tylenchulus semipenetrans* is a devastating pest of citrus causing damage to about 8–12% of citrus species; however, higher infection rates (53–89%) have been observed on citrus in Florida [31]. This nematode life cycle has the second-stage juvenile (J2) as the most infective stage. These nematodes are attracted to citrus roots that have been parasitized by weevil larvae (*D. abbreviatus*) compared to non-parasitized plants [26]. In their experiment, the response of four entomopathogenic nematodes (*S. diaprepesi, S. carpocapsae, S. riobrave,* and *Heterorhabditis indica*) and a plant-parasitic nematode (*T. semipenetrans*) to *D. abbreviatus* parasitism on citrus root stocks (*Poncirus trifoliata, S. citrumelo-* (*C. paradisi* × *P. trifoliata*), and *Citrus aurantium*) was investigated. Results revealed high nematode numbers that moved toward *S. citrumelo* weevil-infested roots, compared to the non-infested ones in spite of the foraging strategy implored by the nematode-foraging strategy and its trophic status. Further, parasitism or non-parasitism of *D. abbreviatus* on the citrus parent line *P. trifoliata* did not influence the attraction level of nematodes, because the nematode responses to the root stock were similar. Production of the volatile, pregeijerene was released after feeding activity by *D. abbreviatus* only within the root zone and absent in the upper portions of shoots. Feeding activity by the adult beetle (*D. abbreviatus*) on the shoots did not stimulate the production of pregeijerene; however, limonene was released. Within the *P. trifoliata* roots, pregeijerene was released; however, the feeding activity of *D. abbreviatus* had no influence in its production.

Maize root volatiles can be associated with the ability of entomopathogenic nematodes in controlling the western corn rootworm. The roots of maize release the volatile (*E*)-β-caryophyllene (EβC) after parasitism by the larvae of *Diabrotica virgifera virgifera*. This chemical, which is a sesquiterpene, serves as an attractant to some species of entomopathogenic nematodes [29, 32, 33]. The volatile (*E*)-β-caryophyllene (EβC) was investigated on the EPN *H. bacteriophora, H. megidis, and S. feltiae* against *D. v. virgifera* larvae in southern Hungary. The maize variety that released (*E*)-β-caryophyllene (EβC) was protected from *H. megidis* and *S. feltiae*.

The roots of cotton (*Gossypium herbaceum*) also emit terpenoid volatiles after the feeding activity of the larvae of the chrysomelid beetle *D. balteata* [25]. This sesquiterpenoid aristolene may be a useful volatile for attraction of the nematode *H. megidis*.

3. Root exudates and nematode control

Plant root exudates and their impact on root-knot nematode egg hatchability are an important development for nematode management. The chemicals within root exudates may either attract or repel nematodes to their host roots. There is experimental evidence to show the influence of root exudates on nematode egg hatch [34–36]. There are specific signals which are generated from exudates of roots; these enable nematodes to be attracted to their hosts. Known compounds that attract second-stage juveniles to host roots include tannic acids, flavonoids, glycoside, fatty acids, and volatile organic molecules [37, 38]. Semiochemicals, for example, small lipophilic molecules produced from root exudates of tomato and rice, enable stylet movement into host cells [39].

Root exudates have within them organic acids and sugars which are generated from mycorrhizal and non-mycorrhizal plants [8]. Flavonoids [40], phenolic compounds [41], amino acids [42], and the plant hormone strigolactone [43] are also constituents of root exudates. Root exudates released by mycorrhizal plants have the potential of attracting *Pseudomonas fluorescens* [44] and the fungus *Trichoderma* spp. [45], both organisms poses nematicidal properties for biocontrol of nematodes [46, 47]. Tomato plants, which formed symbiosis with *Funneliformis mosseae*, had low juvenile numbers of *M. incognita* compared to control plots [48].

In a recent study, the impact of tomato root exudates on *M. incognita* was investigated. These exudates were obtained from the root stocks Baliya (highly resistant, HR), RS2 (moderately resistant, MR), and L-402 (highly susceptible, T). These had varying impacts on *M. incognita* egg hatch and the movements of the second-stage juveniles (J2) [49]. The various root exudates obtained from the tomato root stocks (HR, MR, and T strains) decreased *M. incognita* egg hatchability; furthermore, populations of J2 decreased with the highest mortality rate associated with exudates from the HR plants. There was a much higher repelling rate from the HR genotypes to *M. incognita* J2 compared to the other genotypes. However, exudates from the susceptible genotype (T) attracted the juveniles. *The root exudates are made up of varying constituents from the different AMF species* [50]. Microbial diversity occurring within soils is positively influenced by root exudates [51], and AMF in soils may also produce high facultative anaerobic bacteria, for example, *Streptomyces* species, and actinomycetes [52–54].

4. Soil bacteria and nematode control

Nematodes in soil are subject to infections by bacteria and fungi. This creates the possibility of using soil bacteria to control PPN [55–57]. An effective natural enemy of nematodes is nematophagous bacteria which are ubiquitous with wide host ranges. These organisms have been isolated from soil, plant tissues, cysts, and eggs of nematodes. They directly suppress the activities of nematodes through the production of antibiotics, toxins, as well as enzymes; they also compete for nutrients and space through parasitizing, and therefore provide systemic resistance for plant growth. Their activities promote plant growth though facilitating rhizosphere colonization and enhanced microbial antagonism. Antagonism may be direct, which might result from physical contact, or indirect, which includes activities that do not involve sensing or targeting the PPN. Nematophagous bacteria may be grouped into parasitic and non-parasitic bacteria, opportunistic parasitic bacteria, rhizobacteria, Cry protein-forming bacteria, endophytic bacteria, and symbiotic bacteria based on their mode of parasitism [58].

Biocontrol agents, for example, *Agrobacterium, Alcaligenes, Bacillus, Clostridium, Desulfovibrio, Pseudomonas, Serratia, Streptomyces,* and *Pasteuria penetrans* have potentials for nematode control, have shown great potential for the biological control of nematodes [59, 60]. Nematophagous bacteria affect nematodes by the following modes of action: parasitizing; producing toxins, antibiotics, or enzymes; interfering with nematode-plant-host recognition; competing for nutrients; inducing systemic resistance of plants; and promoting plant health [58].

Among microorganisms occurring in soil, only few have been identified as biocontrol agents for phytonematodes, and some species of fungi and bacteria are the most common parasites of nematodes [57]. Some bacteria are potent antagonists of phytonematodes, and currently some have been developed into commercial bionematicides which are being used to control on the field mainly in advanced countries [61] (**Table 1**). These nematophagous bacteria can be categorized into two groups based on their mechanisms of infection: (i) bacteria that are pathogenic to nematodes or nematode diseases producing bacteria and (ii) bacteria whose secretions or metabolic products are harmful to nematodes or the nematode toxin-producing bacteria. The genus *Pasteuria* are endospore forming which are parasites of nematodes and water fleas [62, 63]. The control of most economically important genera of phytonematodes using nematophagous bacteria has been associated with this genus—*Pasteuria*. The other group includes strains of *Agrobacterium radiobacter, Azotobacter chroococcum, Bacillus* spp., *Clostridium* spp., and *Streptomyces* spp.

Actinobacteria are a group of soil bacteria of importance as biocontrol agents with nematicidal properties [64–67]. The diversity and biocontrol ability of nematicidal actinobacteria have been investigated [67]. In their study, 200 soil samples were obtained from 20 provinces within China. Results revealed 4000 actinobacteria, and these isolates 533 (13.3%) and 488 (12.2%) have some nematicidal activities on the nematodes *Panagrellus redivivus* and *Bursaphelenchus xylophilus,* respectively. Actinobacteria are generally Gram positive bacteria, and have G+C content of >55%. There has been over 70% of bioactive compounds released by these microorganisms with their usage in agriculture and pharmaceutical industry. These organisms release lytic enzymes, and secondary metabolites. One group of metabolites are avermectins which are produced by *S. avermitilis* [68]. Avermectins are useful for nematode control [69]. A previous screen of 502 actinobacteria showed 15 of these with nematicidal impact on *P. redivivus,* a free-living nematode [65].

Streptomyces isolate (CR-43) from Costa Rica had inhibitory impacts on *C. elegans* after a laboratory experimentation [69]. Other studies conducted in the greenhouse showed CR-43 with the potential of reducing root galls on tomato inoculated with *M. incognita.* Furthermore, field studies in Puerto Rico revealed pepper and tomato plants that received CR-43 as treatments having the least gall numbers compared to controls. In an in vitro investigation, *Streptomyces* sp. (CMU-MH021), which is an actinomycete isolated from nematode-infested soils in Thailand, showed the release of secondary metabolites which prevented *M. incognita* egg hatch, and also a decrease in juvenile numbers [70]. The nematicidal properties of various culture filtrates were explored. The modified basal (MB) medium gave the highest activity against *M. incognita.* The broth microdilution technique was applied for understanding the nematicidal activity of fervenulin. Inhibitory concentrations for both egg hatch (30 μg/ml)

Product name	Microbial origin	Company or institution	Country	Nematode target	References
Econem	*Pasteuria usgae* (or *P. penetrans)*	Bayer Crop Science	Multinational	Sting (or root knot)	[76]
Avid 0.15EC (orAbamectin	*Bacillus thuringensis*	Syngenta Group company	Multinational	Root-knot and other nematodes	[190]
Bionem-WP, BioSafe-WP, and Chancellor-WP	*B. armus*	Agro Green	Multinational	Root-knot and other nematodes including	[190]
Nortica VOTIVO PONCHO/ VOTIVO	*B. armus*	Bayer CropScience	Multinational	*Heterodera avenae*	[76]
Deny Blue circle	*Burkholderia capacia*	Stine Microbial Wisconsin Products	USA	*Meloidogyne incognita*	[191]
Biostart®	*Bacillus subtilis*	Bio-Cat	USA	Root knot nematodes	[192]
BiostartL™	*B. laterosporus, B. ncheniformis* (mixture)	Rhcon-Vltova			
Nemix	*Bacillus subtilis, B. ncheniformis*	AgriLife/Chr. Hansen	Brazil		[192]
Nemaless	*Serrata marcescens*	Agricultural Research Centre	Giza, Egypt	Root-knot and other phytonematode	[193]
SHEATHGUARD (or Sudozone)	*Pseudomonas, P. fluorescens*	Agri Life (Ind Limited or Agri Land Biotech)	Hyderabad,India	Nematode such as root-knot,cyst and Citrus nematode	http:www. agrilife.in/ biopestl_ microrigin_ sheathguard_ pf.htm
Xlan Mile	*Bacillus cereus*	XlnYlZhong kai Agro-Chemical Industry Co., ltd	China	*Meloidogyne* spp. on vegetables	[194]
Pathway Consortia®	*Bacillus* spp. *Trichoderma* spp., *P. flurescens, Streptomyces* spp.	Pathway Holdings	USA	Phytonematodes	[1]
Micronema	*Bacillus* sp., *Pseudomonas* sp., *Rhizobacterium* sp., *Rhizobium* sp.	Agricultural Research Centre	Giza, Egypt	Root-knot and other phytonematodes	[195]

CAB International 2015. *Biocontrol Agents of Phytonematodes* (eds T.H. Askary and P.R.P. Martinelli)

Table 1. Commercial products of bacteria for phytonematode control.

and *M. incognita* juvenile mortality (120 μg/ml) were noted. An evaluation of both *in vitro* and *in vivo* nematicidal potential of extracts from *S. hydrogenans* strain DH16 against *M. incognita* prevented egg hatch (>95%) and a high mortality rate (95%) of juveniles after 96 h [71].

Furthermore, two compounds [10-(2,2-dimethyl-cyclohexyl)-6,9-dihydroxy-4,9-dimethyl-dec-2-enoic acid methyl ester] purified from the streptomycete were evaluated for their efficacy against *M. incognita*. The juvenile nematode mortality varied with the concentration rates with high mortality observed at high concentrations, for example, a concentration of 100 μg/ml caused 95% mortality after 96 h.

The marine bacteria *B. firmus* strain YBf-10 shows its efficacy as a biocontrol agent on *M. incognita* (eggs and juveniles) through a systemic action [72]. The application of this strain through drenching of tomato plants inoculated with *M. incognita* produced plants with reduced galls and egg masses, and nematode numbers in soil samples.

Pasteuria, which is an endospore-forming bacteria with various species within this genus, may be implored as biocontrol agents and there are four nematode antagonists within this genus. Among these, *P. penetrans, P. thornei, P. nishizawae,* and *P. usgae* are parasites on root-knot nematodes, lesion nematodes [73], and *Belonolaimus* spp. [74]. Commercialization of *Pasteuria* products for nematode control is, however, limited by two factors: (i) a narrow host range [75] and (ii) growth *in vitro* is slow and production is tedious [76]. *In vitro* production of *Pasteuria* spp. was initiated after *Pasteuria.* Bioscience Alachua (Florida, USA) filed a patent in 2004, for the production of the product Econem™, a product which is target-specific and has been designed to control sting nematodes (*Belonolaimus* spp.) in turf.

5. Fungi and symbiotic reprogramming in host cells

Arbuscular mycorrhiza fungi (AMF) are in the phylum Glomeromycota [77]; these fungi form symbiotic associations with plant roots and provide phosphorus, nitrogen, and water to plants [78]. Another advantage derived from this association is tolerance to biotic and abiotic stresses by host plants [79, 80]. Native strains of AMF are used as bio-fertilizers for enhanced plant growth, including root and tuber crops and for nematode management [81, 82]. The AMF releases signal that are transmitted systemically and these are to target non-infected parts of roots [83, 84].Within the soil microbes with beneficial properties, for example, AMF are recognized by plants as invaders leading to the triggering of an immune response (**Figure 1A**) [85], and this signaling is associated with microbe-associated molecular patterns (MAMPs), which further induce MAMP-triggered immunity (MTI) [86, 87]. Second, there symbiotic activities within cells can be activated through mycorrhizal Myc factors if perceived (**Figure 1B**). The SP7 effector within the AMF *Glomus intraradices* is a characteristic defense signal in the fungi [88], and its expression occurs in host roots [85].

Plant cells with roots undergo reprogramming activities for successful establishment of symbiosis with symbionts (e.g., arbuscular mycorrhizal (AM) and root-nodule (RN) symbiosis) [89] (**Figure 2B**). However, this reprogramming phenomenon is absent in an asymbiotic root

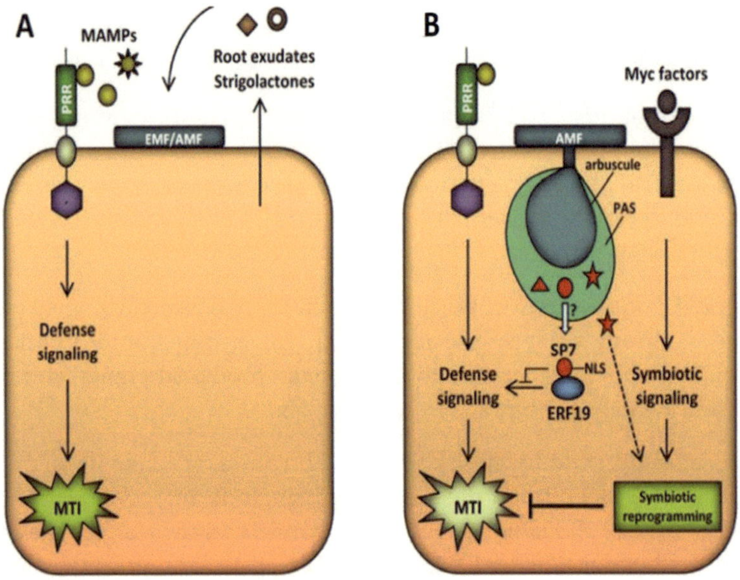

Figure 1. Model for the modulation of host immunity in ectomycorrhizal (EMF) and arbuscular mycorrhizal (AMF) fungi. (A) Root exudates recruit symbiotic mycorrhizal fungi and prime them for the interaction. Host plants initially recognize ectomycorrhizal (EMF) and arbuscular mycorrhizal (AMF) fungi as potential invaders; pattern recognition receptors (PRR) in the host perceive microbe-associated molecular patterns (MAMPs) and a signaling cascade is initiated that results in MAMP-triggered immunity (MTI). (B) The establishment of the symbiotic program in plant cells, which is activated upon perception of the mycorrhizal Myc factors, counteracts MTI with mechanisms yet to be defined. Molecules secreted in the apoplastic or peri-arbuscular space (PAS) may act as either apoplastic or cytoplasmic effectors to suppress the MTI response or promote the symbiotic program. The AMF *Glomus intraradices* secretes the SP7 effector which is translocated into the plant cytosol; a nuclear localization signal (NLS) targets SP7 to the nucleus, where it interacts with the defense-related transcription factor ERF19 to block the ERF19-mediated transcriptional program [85].

cell (**Figure 1B**). Within the soil, roots of plants continuously produce and release root exudates and strigolactines as observed in an asymbiotic root cell. Signals are transmitted to the nucleus through transcription factors, gene expression occurs, and there is cell-to-cell communication. There are also plant receptors within the root cells that detect mineral concentration in soils. In a root cell that either interacts with AM or RN fungi, there is release of both flavonoids and strigolactones, two factors (Nod and Myc) are released from the symbionts and these turn on the calcium spiking. Within the RN symbiosis, flavonoids from the plant root turn on the Nod transcription factor, and enables bacteria to produce lipochitooligosaccharide nod factors. These Nod factors stimulate root-nodule development, which are needed by rhizobia. Strigolactones further stimulate AM fungi and hyphal branching occurs [90]. The root cortex is usually colonized by AM fungi and produces substantial hyphae (arbuscules). During the development of the arbuscle, it becomes enveloped within the peri-arbuscular membrane (PAM), and essential proteins are moved to the plant cell within the PAM [91]. Jasmonic acid (JA) and methyl jasmonate (MeJA) can stimulate the expression of Nod genes [92] and release of Nod factors [93], in rhizobia after their application exogenously.

http://dx.doi.org/10.5772/intechopen.69164

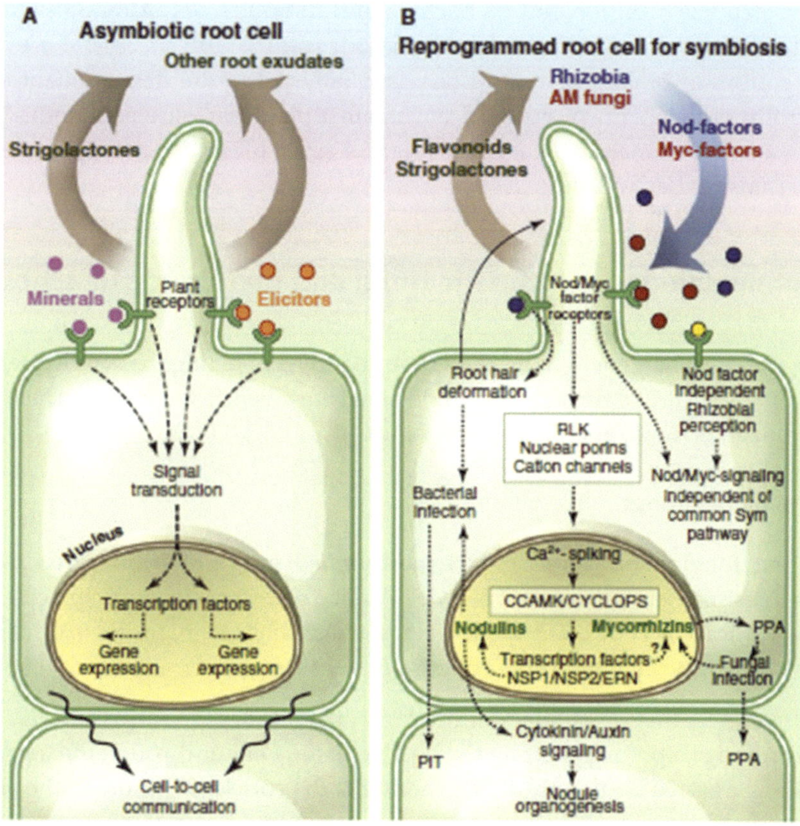

Figure 2. Signal exchange during symbiosis. (A) An asymbiotic cell constitutively releases root exudates, including strigolactones. The root cell monitors the concentration of minerals and microbial organisms in the soil and transduces the respective signals. Integration of the signals occurs at the cellular and organismic levels and includes cell-to-cell communication. (B) A root-hair cell primed for interaction with rhizobia or AM fungi, respectively. Plant roots release flavonoids and strigolactones that prime the rhizobia and AM fungi. Nod and Myc factors act as signals from the symbionts to plant root cells that activate calcium spiking via the Sym pathway (boxed). The potential differential activation of CaMK/Cyclops leads to differential induction of nodulation-specific transcription factors (NSP1, NSP2, and ERN) and unknown mycorrhizal-specific transcription factors. Rhizobial and mycorrhizal infection require the common Sym pathway but also exhibit recognition and signaling independent of this pathway. The path for fungal infection and the IT is predicted by the PiT and the PPA, respectively, indicating directed signaling to neighboring cells. Nodule organogenesis is induced in inner cortical cells after nod-factor perception by epidermal cells. This requires cytokinin signaling and is associated with changes in auxin levels [89].

6. Fungi antagonists of nematodes

Biological control, defined as the management of plant diseases and pests by means of other living organisms, mainly concerns the exploitation of microbial agents [94]. Under natural conditions, biocontrol agents that are associated with plant-parasitic nematodes usually exist [95]. These organisms act through parasitism, predation, antagonism, or competition [96], but their successful activity depends on a number of parameters, including soil environmental factors [97]. Many beneficial organisms were found to attack plant-parasitic nematodes but most research has been focused on bacteria and fungi [94, 98]. Although few biological agents had been until recently adopted for nematode control with successful use, the current progress in studies of biological control has gradually led to the development of commercial biocontrol products with proven efficacy against plant-parasitic nematodes. Studies on fungal antagonists of nematodes have been started since 1874 with the first observations of *Harposporium anguillulae,* by Lohde.

7. Types of nematode-antagonistic fungi and their mode of action

Species of several fungal genera have been reported to have biological activity against plant-parasitic nematodes [58]. Hallmann et al. [98] classified these beneficial fungi into nematophagous fungi, saprophagous fungi, and endophytic fungi.

7.1. Nematophagous fungi

Nematophagous fungi are the largest and the most studied group of the fungi involved in the biological control against plant-parasitic nematodes. Among nematophagous fungi, which have been tested for their efficacy in controlling nematodes, some are obligate parasites (e.g., *Nematophthora gynophila*), others are facultative or opportunistic parasites (e.g., *Pochonia chlamydosporia*) [98].

Obligate parasites require a residual population of nematodes for their survival. Infection is initiated when fungal spores penetrate the host nematode either through the gastrointestinal tract after being ingested or directly after adhering to the cuticle [98]. Among the obligate fungal parasites, *Hirsutella* spp. and *Drechmeria coniospora* have shown to be interesting in terms of their biology, mode of action, and nematode control potential. Infection of these fungi is initiated by the adhesion of small conidia to the nematode cuticle. However, obligate parasites are difficult to grow in culture.

The facultative parasites are able to switch between saprophytic state in soil and rhizosphere into parasites that infect nematodes, depending on environmental circumstances. Nematode infection occurs either by way of adhesives spores or by trapping structures, or through an appressorium [94]. Depending on their mode of action, nematophagous fungi can attack nematodes during all stages of their life cycle.

In addition to the fungi described above, some form a mycelium able to capture plant-parasitic nematodes. They are called predacious fungi or nematode-trapping fungi and act through different trapping structures including fungal hyphae covered with adhesive secretions (e.g., *Stylopage* spp.), adhesive branches (e.g., *Monacrosporium cionopagum*), adhesive spores (*Meristacrum* spp.), or adhesive knobs (*Arthrobotrys* spp., *Nematoctonus* spp.) [99, 100]. These fungi also produce nematicidal compounds such as linoleic acid (e.g., *A. oligospora*) or pleurotin (e.g., *N. robustus*) [101].

7.2. Saprophagous fungi

Among the saprophagous fungi present in the bulk soil, some have been reported to be antagonistic toward plant-parasitic nematodes. This group was represented by the genus

Trichoderma, a ubiquitous soil fungus that also colonizes the root surface and cortex [98]. *Trichoderma* spp. was first reported to be parasite of other fungi [102], before being identified as an antagonist of plant-parasitic nematodes [103, 104]. A number of *Trichoderma* species, for example, *T. asperellum, T. hamatum, harzianum,* and *T. viride,* were reported to infect eggs and juveniles of root-knot nematodes [105, 106]. Several possible mechanisms including the production of antifungal metabolites, competition for space and nutrients, mycoparasitism, plant growth promotion, and induction of the defense responses in plants have been suggested as mechanisms for their biocontrol activity [107, 108]. Other saprophagous fungi with antagonistic activity against plant-parasitic nematodes include species of the genus *Gliocladium, Acremonium,* and *Cylindrocarpon* [109–111].

7.3. Endophytic fungi

Endophytic fungi have been considered as important fungi in the biological control of plant-parasitic nematodes. The implication of endophytic fungi in root-knot nematode reduction was first demonstrated with arbuscular mycorrhizal fungi on vegetables [112].

AMFs are obligate fungi, which form symbiotic associations with numerous plant species, with the primary function of improving plant nutrient uptake [113]. Arbuscular mycorrhizal fungi are obligate plant symbionts. According to Harley and Smith [114], AMFs establish with their host plant an interdependent mutualistic relationship (symbiosis) where the host plant receives mineral nutrients, while the fungus obtains photosynthesis-derived carbon compounds from the plant [115]. Three major types of mycorrhizal associations—ectomycorrhiza, endomycorrhiza, and ectomycorrhizal—endomycorrhizal intermediate type—have been distinguished [116]. Their endophytic nature enables associated (infected) plants to overcome biotic [117] and abiotic stresses [118]. Potential modes of actions developed by AMF during the protective activity against plant pathogens reviewed by Whipps [119] include (1) the direct competition or inhibition, (2) enhanced or altered plant growth, morphology, and nutrition, (3) biochemical changes associated with plant defense mechanisms and induced resistance, and (4) development of an antagonistic microbiota. Other studies have recently reported the ability of AMF to induce systemic resistance against plant-parasitic nematodes in the root system [120].

Another important endophytic fungus in nematode control but with saprophytic nature is the non-pathogenic *Fusarium* species, *Fusarium oxysporum*. Reduction of nematode penetration into the host plant root and induction of systemic resistance to plants have been considered as the main mechanisms by which *F. oxyporum* reduced nematode parasitism [121–123].

8. Potential of antagonistic fungi in nematode control

A large number of fungi have been tested for their potential as biological control agents of plant-parasitic nematodes. Until recently, few had been adopted for nematode control with successful use [98]. However, the current progress in studies of biological control has gradually led to the development of commercial biocontrol products with proven efficacy against plant-parasitic nematodes. In this section, most fungal studies will be discussed.

8.1. P. chlamydosporia

Species of *Pochonia* are widely distributed in agricultural soils and infect eggs of plant-parasitic nematodes, snails, and slugs [96].

Within the genus *Pochonia, P. chlamydosporia* appears the most effective in infecting nematode eggs [124]. *P. chlamydosporia* includes two subspecies *P. chlamydosporia var. chlamydosporia* and *P. chlamydosporia var. catenulatum* [125] which are considered non-pathogenic to plants, higher animals, and humans [126]. This species is one of the major facultative antagonistic fungi that can parasitize egg and female stages of root-knot nematodes and female cyst nematodes [96, 127, 128]. Parasitism of this fungus is based on appressorial formation developed from undifferentiated hyphae, which allows the colonization of the egg surface and penetration through both mechanical and enzymatic actions [129]. Observations during the infection process have shown that the penetration of the eggshell occurs from both the appressorium and the lateral branch of the mycelium, and leads to the disintegration and the dissolution of three layers composing the eggshell: the vitelline layer, chitin layer, and lipoprotein layer [130, 131]. The infection process is affected by the nematode host [130], suggesting that fungal growth, development, and penetration of the eggshell may be influenced by signals from the eggs [132]. Different enzymes, in particular proteases and chitinases, are important for the infection processes, and VCP1 proteases being the most known proteases with enzymatic activity against the nematode eggshells [94, 130].

The efficacy of *P. chlamydosporia* has been reported to be affected by three key factors: the fungal density in the rhizosphere, the rate of egg development in the egg masses, and the size of the galls in which the female nematodes develop [133]. *P. chlamydosporia* is found to be more abundant in the rhizosphere and on nematode-infected roots, and parasitism may promote the long-term survival of the fungus in soil [96]. However, the extent of colonization depends on the fungus isolate and the plant species [134, 135]. Although isolates of *P. chlamydosporia* differ significantly in their ability to parasitize the eggs of different nematode species, they have shown little host specificity [136].

Formulations based on *P. chlamydosporia* have been developed and are currently being commercialized (e.g., KlamiC® based on *P. chlamydosporia* var. *catenulata* RES 392 from Cuba) [98, 137].

8.2. *Trichoderma* spp

Species of *Trichoderma* are ubiquitous soil-borne fungi that can colonize the root surface as well as the cortex [138, 139]. Several species of *Trichoderma* have been considered for biocontrol of plant-parasitic nematodes [104]. Some species were found to be associated with eggs of root-knot nematodes in vegetable fields [106].

Against nematodes, *Trichoderma* spp. can provide excellent control and are viewed as strong contenders for development as biocontrol agents [104]. In various studies, species of *Trichoderma* were reported to show antagonistic activity against eggs and juveniles of root-knot nematodes in *in vitro* conditions [105] and to infect nematode egg masses and reduce juvenile populations in non-sterilized field soil [140]. *Trichoderma* spp. were shown to efficiently control root-knot nematodes when they were applied before planting [104, 141]. Methods suggested for their application include seed treatment, dry formulation, or soil drench [98]. However, isolates of the same species of *Trichoderma* can differ markedly in their rhizosphere competence, biocontrol potential toward nematodes, and plant growth promotion [141].

Different mechanisms have been suggested as mechanisms developed by *Trichoderma* against nematodes. The first observable interaction between *Trichoderma* spp. and its host is expressed by direct growth of the mycoparasite hyphae initiated by a chemotropic reaction toward the host [105]. The hyphae, upon contact, coil around and penetrate the host. This process involves the release of lytic enzymes by *Trichoderma* spp. [142], which serves to partially degrade the host cell wall. Lytic enzymes such as chitinases, glucanases, and proteases, seem to be particularly important in the mycoparasitic process. Induction of defense responses in plants by *Trichoderma* spp. was also observed through increased peroxidase and chitinase activities following fungal inoculation and a strengthening of the epidermal and cortical cell walls as the deposition of newly formed barriers [143]. These authors also reported increased enzyme activities in the leaves, suggesting a systemic defense response to the presence of *Trichoderma* in the rhizosphere. When monitoring fungus-nematode interactions, Sharon et al. [105] observed that in pre-inoculated soil, the fungus colonizing the roots interacts with the penetrating juveniles and colonizes their penetration sites, indicating also a competition for spaces. *Trichoderma*-based products are commercially available and used to control plant-parasitic nematodes on different crops. Successful examples include BioNem® [144] and T-22™ Planter Box [145].

9. Arbuscular mycorrhizal fungi

A number of studies have demonstrated the contribution of arbuscular mycorrhizal fungi in improving soil structure [146], plant mineral uptake, and plant growth [113, 147, 148] enhancing plant tolerance to pollution with toxic metals [149, 150], resistance to drought stress [151], and reducing the effect of plant diseases [117, 152–154]. AMFs have also been reported to protect host plants against plant-parasitic nematodes [81, 98, 155]. The interaction between AMF-colonized plants and plant-parasitic nematodes has been reviewed by several authors [98, 156, 157]. AMFs have also been shown to suppress the effect of damage [112, 158], although some studies have shown no effects against these pests [159, 160]. However, the efficacy of AMF against nematodes may be influenced by a number of factors including prevailing environmental conditions [161], cultivar [159], nutrient status of the field [162], and the timing of application [163]. Existing knowledge suggests the application of the fungi in the nursery or to introduce suitable mycorrhizal crops into the rotation pattern for efficient pest control [98]. Pre-inoculation of seedlings with AMF, for example, has resulted in high levels of root colonization, followed by a significant reduction of nematode infection [164]. However, recent studies showed that the level of reduction of RKN was not necessarily dependent on high-root mycorrhization, while the interaction between crop cultivar-AMF strains is also important [165]. Furthermore, direct inoculation of AMF inoculum into the transplanting hole prior to planting may provide plant protection against root-knot nematodes, indicating possible use of AMF for seed-growing crops [165]. Some studies on the combination of AMF with other antagonists have provided promising clues for their successful integration into nematode control strategies [166, 167]. Different formulations based on AMF strains (e.g., *F. mosseae*- and *G. dussii*-based products from BIORIZE© in Dijon, France) were commercially developed for use in crop protection against plant-parasitic nematodes [81, 165].

9.1. Paecilomyces lilacinus

Paecilomyces lilacinus (Thom) Samson seems to be most frequent in warmer regions, although it has been reported in different parts of the world and from various habitats [126, 168]. Investigations on the biocontrol activity of the fungus toward plant-parasitic nematodes started after Jatala et al. [169] discovered infection of eggs and females of *M. incognita* and eggs of *Globodera pallida*. Both mechanical and enzymatic activities may be involved in the host penetration. *P. lilacinus* first colonizes the gelatinous matrix of *Meloidgyne, Tylenchulus,* and *Naccobus,* and cysts of cyst nematodes, develops a mycelium network, then engulfs and penetrates the nematode eggs through an appressorium or simple hyphae [126, 169]. Following penetration, the fungus grows on the early embryonic development, depletes all nutrients in the eggs, breaks the cuticle of the infected egg and infects other eggs. Although *P. lilacinus* is considered as egg-pathogenic fungus, Holland et al. [170] observed in *in vitro* experiment infection of third- and fourth-stage juveniles and adult females of *M. javanica.*

P. lilacinus is among the most widely studied microorganisms used for the management of plant-parasitic nematodes. Its success in controlling plant-parasitic nematodes has led to the development of commercial products such as MeloCon® WG by Bayer in Germany and PAECILO® by AgriLife in India [171].

9.2. Fusarium oxysporum

The interest in the non-pathogenic *Fusarium oxysporum* for nematode control is stimulated after several isolates were reported to reduce the banana root rotting caused by *Pratylenchus goodeyi* [172]. This endophytic fungus was reported as the most abundant endophytes of banana (*Musa* spp.), for example, in Uganda [173, 174]. In various studies, the strain *F. oxysporum* FO162 has shown the ability to reduce penetration of damage caused by plant-parasitic nematodes on tomato and banana [175–178]. Dababat and Sikora [123] reported that plants colonized by *F. oxyporum* were less attractive or exuded substances that were repellent toward nematodes. The endophytic fungus can infect nematodes at any stages and reduce significantly the plant damage [121, 179]. Recent studies indicate that the non-pathogenic *F. oxysporum* is a successful biocontrol agent for plant-parasitic nematodes with positive effect on the plant growth [180].

9.3. *Arthrobotrys* spp

Arthrobotrys species are trapping fungi which immobilize nematodes [189] using different trap structures [181]. The species *A. oligospora* was the first recognized nematode-trapping fungus [182]. *A. conoides* and *A. oligospora* makes three-dimensional adhesive network to trap soil-inhabiting nematodes [94, 183]. *A. candida* usually forms non-constructing rings [184] but Al kader [181] reported a formation of adhesive hyphae capturing nematodes and then trophic hyphae within nematodes' body to digest nematode contents. *A. brochopaga* forms ring traps that constrict around the body of a nematode passing through them [185]. The presence of the nematode is important in the initiation of the trapping structures [186]. Nematode species did not affect the type of trap structure but most probably the quantity of these traps. Santos et al. [187] reported substantial variability in virulence among isolates of the same species. Host recognition and adhesion by the fungus were the first steps in the infection of the host nematode. This recognition has been attributed to a molecular interaction of certain proteins on the fungal surface with sugar molecules on the nematode cuticle [183]. Substantial variability in virulence among isolates of the same species was observed [187]. Nordbring-Hertz et al. [188] reported that *Aphelenchus avenae* can avoid to be captured by the fungi structures, especially for the young nematode.

10. Conclusions

Beneficial microbial inocula can be applied for large-scale field management of nematodes which will result in increased yields. However, further research into the various biocontrol measures used by organisms is necessary, and this can be achieved through genomic approaches; this will enhance understanding of the various complex mechanisms used by these organisms on nematodes. Strains of these organisms may be effective in their local occurrences, and therefore countrywide surveys of soils will enable location-specific strains to be isolated and characterized. These local strains once characterized can be produced in large quantities and distributed to farmers for applications in their fields.

Author details

Seloame Tatu Nyaku[1,2*], Antoine Affokpon[3], Agyemang Danquah[1,2] and Francis Collison Brentu[4]

*Address all correspondence to: seloame.nyaku@gmail.com

1 Department of Crop Science, College of Basic and Applied Sciences, University of Ghana, Legon-Accra, Ghana

2 West Africa Centre for Crop Improvement (WACCI), College of Basic and Applied Sciences (CBAS) University of Ghana (UG), Legon, Ghana

3 Faculty of Agronomic Sciences, School of Plant Sciences, University of Abomey-Calavi, Cotonou, Benin

4 Forest and Horticultural Crops Research Centre (FOHCREC), College of Basic and Applied Sciences, University of Ghana, Kade, Ghana

References

[1] Abd-Elgawad MM, Askary TH. Impact of phytonematodes on agriculture economy. In: Askary TH, Martinelli PRP, editors. Biocontrol Agents of Phytonematodes. Wallingford, UK: CAB International; 2015. pp. 3-49

[2] Stirling GR. Biological Control of Plant Parasitic Nematode: Progress, Problems and Prospects. Wallington, UK: CAB International; 1991. p. 282

[3] Abd-Elgawad MM. Biological control agents of plant-parasitic nematodes. Egyptian Journal of Biological Pest Control. 2016;**26**:423-429

[4] Effmert U, Buss D, Rohrbeck D, Piechulla B. Localization of the synthesis and emission of scent compounds within the Xower. In: Dudareva N, Pichersky E, editors. Floral Scents. London: CRC Press Taylor and Francis Group; 2006. pp 105-124

[5] Aochi YO, Farmer WJ. Impact of soil microstructure on the molecular transport dynamics of 1, 2-dichlorethane. Geoderma. 2005;**127**:137-153

[6] Barber DA, Martin JK. The release of organic substances by cereal roots into soil. New Phytology. 1976;**76**:69-80

[7] Roshchina VV, Roshchina VD. The Excretory Function of Higher Plants. Berlin: Springer; 1993. p. 314. doi: 10.1007/978-3-642-78130-8

[8] Hage-Ahmed K, Moyses A, Voglgruber A, Hadacek F, Steinkellner S. Alterations in root exudation of intercropped tomato mediated by the arbuscular mycorrhizal fungus *Glomus mosseae* and the soilborne pathogen *Fusarium oxysporum* f. sp. lycopersici. Journal of Phytopathology. 2013;**161**:763-773. doi:10.1111/jph.12130

[9] Lewis EE, Campbell JF, Griffin C, Kaya HK, Peters A. Behavioral ecology of entomopathogenic nematodes. Biological Control. 2006;**38**:66-79

[10] Pline M, Dusenbery DB. Responses of plant-parasitic nematode *Meloidogyne incognita* to carbon dioxide determined by video camera-computer tracking. Journal of Chemical Ecology. 1987;**13**(4):873-888. doi: 10.1007/BF01020167 PMID: 24302053

[11] Dusenbery DB. Theoretical range over which bacteria and nematodes could use carbon dioxide to locate plant roots. Journal of Chemical Ecology. 1987;**13**:1617-1624

[12] Klinger J. Die Orientierung von *Ditylenchus dipsaci* in gemessenen künstlichen und biologischen CO2-Gradienten. Nematologica. 1963;**9**:185-199

[13] Bauske EM, Rodríguez-Kábana R, Estaun V, Kloepper JW, Robertson DG, Weaver CF, King PS. Management of *Meloidogyne incognita* on cotton by use of botanical aromatic compounds. Nematropica. 1994;**24**:143-150

[14] Oka Y, Nacar S, Putievsky E, Ravid U, Yaniv Z, Spiegel Y. Nematicidal activity of essential oils and their components against the root-knot nematode. Phytopathology. 2000; **90**:710-715

[15] Rohlof J. Volatiles from rhizomes of *Rhodiola rosea* L. Phytochemistry. 2002;**59**:655-661

[16] Kokalis-Burelle N, Martinez-Ochoa N, Rodríguez-Kabana R, Kloepper JW. Development of multi-component transplant mixes for suppression of *Meloidogyne incognita* on tomato (*Lycopersicum esculentum*). Journal of Nematology. 2002;**34**:362-369

[17] Bertoli A, Pistelli L, Morelli I, Fraternale D, Giamperi L, Ricci D. Volatile constituents of different parts (roots, stems, and leaves) of *Smyrnium olusatrum* L. Flavour Fragrance Journal. 2004;**19**:522-525

[18] Weissteiner S, Schütz S. Are different volatile pattern influencing host plant choice of belowground living insects. Mitteilungen der Deutschen Gesellschaft für Allgemeine und Angewandte Entomologie. 2006;**15**:51-55

[19] Turlings TCJ, Tumlinson JH, Lewis WJ. Exploitation of herbivore-induced plant odors by host-seeking parasitic wasps. Science. 1990;**250**:1251-1253

[20] Heil M. Indirect defence via tritrophic interactions. New Phytologist. 2008;**178**:41-61

[21] Dicke M, Baldwin IT. The evolutionary context for herbivore-induced plant volatiles: Beyond the 'cry for help'. Trends in Plant Science. 2010;**15**:167-175

[22] Dicke M, Sabelis MW. How plants obtain predatory mites as bodyguards. Netherlands Journal of Zoology. 1988;**38**:148-165

[23] Alborn HT, Jones TH, Stenhagen GS, Tumlinson JH. Identification and synthesis of volicitin and related components from beet armyworm oral secretions. Journal of Chemical Ecology. 2000;**26**:203-220

[24] Turlings TCJ, Alborn HT, Loughrin JH, Tumlinson JH. Volicitin, an elicitor of maize volatiles in the oral secretion of *Spodoptera exigua*: Its isolation and bio-activity. Journal of Chemical Ecology. 2000;**26**:189-202

[25] Rasmann S, Turlings TCJ. First insights into specificity of belowground tritrophic interactions. Oikos. 2008;**117**:362-369

[26] Ali JG, Alborn HT, Stelinski LL. Constitutive and induced subterranean plant volatiles attract both entomopathogenic and plant-parasitic nematodes. Journal of Ecology. 2011;**99**:26-35

[27] van Tol RWHM, van der Sommen ATC, BoV MIC, van Bezooijen J, Sabelis MW, Smits PH. Plants protect their roots by alerting the enemies of grubs. Ecological Letters. 2001;**4**:292-294

[28] Neveu N, Grandgirard J, Nenon JP, Cortesero AM. Systemic release of herbivore-induced plant volatiles by turnips infested by concealed root-feeding larvae *Delia radicum* L. Journal of Chemical Ecology. 2002;**28**:1717-1732

[29] Rasman S, Köllner TG, Degenhardt J, Hiltpold I, Toepfer S, Kuhlmann U, Gershenzon J, Turlings TCJ. Recruitment of entomopathogenic nematodes by insect-damaged maize roots. Nature. 2005;**434**:732-737

[30] Ali JG, Alborn HT, Stelinski LL. Subterranean herbivore-induced volatiles released by citrus roots attract entomopathogenic nematodes. Journal of Chemical Ecology. 2010;**36**:361-368

[31] Duncan LW, Ferguson JJ, Dunn RA, Noling JW. Application of Taylor's power law to sample statistics of *Tylenchulus semipenetrans* in Florida citrus. Supplement to the Journal of Nematology (Annals of Applied Nematology). 1989;**21**:707-711

[32] Hiltpold I, Toepfer S, Kuhlmann U, Turlings TCJ. How maize root volatiles affect the efficacy of entomopathogenic nematodes in controlling the western corn rootworm. Chemoecology. 2010;**20**:155-162

[33] Degenhardt J, Hiltpold I, Kollner TG, Frey M, Gierl A, Gershenzon J, Hibbard BE, Ellersieck MR, Turlings TCJ. Restoring a maize root signal that attracts insect-killing nematodes to control a major pest. In: Proceedings the National Academy of Sciences United States of America. 2009;**106**:13213-13218

[34] Perry RN, Clarke AJ. Hatching mechanisms of nematodes. Parasitology. 1981;**83**(02):435-449

[35] Curtis RH, Robinson AF, Perry RN. Hatch and Host Location of Root-Knot Nematodes. Wallington, UK: CAB International; 2009. pp. 139-162. 10.1079/9781845934927.0139

[36] Pudasaini MP, Viaene N, Moens M. Hatching of the root-lesion nematode, *Pratylenchus penetrans*, under the influence of temperature and host. Nematology. 2008;**10**(1):47-54

[37] Chitwood DJ. Phytochemical based strategies for nematode control. Annual Review of Phytopathology. 2002;**40**(1):221-249

[38] Rasmann S, Hiltpold I, Ali J. The Role of Root-Produced Volatile Secondary Metabolites in Mediating Soil Interactions, Advances in Selected Plant Physiology Aspects, Montanaro, G, editor. InTech Open Access Publisher; 2012 DOI: 10.5772/34304. Available from: https://www.intechopen.com/books/advances-in-selected-plant-physiology-aspects/the-role-of-root-produced-volatile-secondary-metabolites-in-mediating-soil-interactions

[39] Dutta TK, Powers SJ, Gaur HS, Birkett M, Curtis RH. Effect of small lipophilic molecules in tomato and rice root exudates on the behaviour of *Meloidogyne incognita* and *M. graminicola*. Nematology. 2012;**14**(3):309-320

[40] Steinkellner S, LendzemoV, Langer I, Schweiger P, Khaosaad T, Toussaint J-P, et al. Flavonoids and strigolactones in root exudates as signals in symbiotic and pathogenic plant-fungus interactions. Molecules. 2007;**12**:1290-1306. doi: 10.3390/12071290

[41] McArthur DA, Knowles NR. Resistance responses of potato vesicular-arbuscular mycorrhizal fungi under varying abiotic phosphorus levels. Plant Physiology. 1992;**100**:341-351. doi: 10.1104/pp.100.1.341

[42] Harrier LA, Watson CA. The potential role of arbuscular mycorrhizal (AM) fungi in the bio-protection of plants against soil-borne pathogens in organic and/or other sustainable farming systems. Pest Management Science. 2004;**60**:149-157. doi: 10.1002/ps.820

[43] López-Ráez JA, Charnikhova T, Fernández I, Bouwmeester H, Pozo MJ. Arbuscular mycorrhizal symbiosis decreases strigolactone production in tomato. Journal of Plant Physiology. 2011;**168**:294-297. doi: 10.1016/j.jplph.2010. 08.011

[44] Sood GS. Chemotactic response of plant-growth-promoting bacteria towards roots of vesicular-arbuscular mycorrhizal tomato plants. FEMS Microbiology Ecology. 2003; **45**:219-227. doi: 10.1016/S0168-6496(03)00155-7

[45] Druzhinina IS, Seidl-Seiboth V, Herrera-Estrella A, Horwitz BA, Kenerley CM, Monte E, et al. Trichoderma: The genomics of opportunistic success. Nature Reviews Microbiology. 2011;**9**:749-759. doi: 10.1038/nrmicro2637

[46] Dong LQ, Zhang KQ. Microbial control of plant-parasitic nematodes: A five-party interaction. Plant Soil. 2006;**288**:31-45. doi: 10.1007/s11104-006-9009-3

[47] Sikora RA, Pocasangre L, FeldeZum A, Niere B, Vu TT, Dababat AA. Mutualistic endophytic fungi and in planta suppressiveness to plant-parasitic nematodes. Biological Control. 2008;**46**:15-23. doi: 10.1016/j.biocontrol.2008.02.011

[48] Vos C, Claerhout S, Mkandawire R, Panis B, de Waele D, Elsen A. Arbuscular mycorrhizal fungi reduce root-knot nematode penetration through altered root exudation of their host. Plant Soil. 2012b;354:335-345. 10.1007/s11104-011-1070-x

[49] Yang G, Zhou B, Zhang X, Zhang Z, Wu Y, Zhang Y, et al. Effects of tomato root exudates on *Meloidogyne incognita*. PLoS One. 2016;**11**(4):e0154675. doi: 10.1371/journal.pone.0154675

[50] Kobra N, Jalil K, Youbert G. Effects of three Glomus species as biocontrol agents against *Verticillium*-induced wilt in cotton. Journal of Plant Protection Research. 2009;**49**:185-189. 10.2478/v10045-009-0027-z

[51] Lioussanne L. The role of the arbuscular mycorrhiza-associated rhizobacteria in the biocontrol of soilborne phyto-pathogens. Spanish Journal of Agricultural Research. 2010;**8**:3-5. doi: 10.5424/sjar/201008S1-5301

[52] Scheublin TR, Sanders IR, Keel C, van der Meer JR. Characterisation of microbial communities colonising the hyphal surfaces of arbuscular mycorrhizal fungi. ISMEJ. 2010; **4**:752-763. doi: 10.1038/ismej. 2010.5

[53] Miransari M. Interactions between arbuscular mycorrhizal fungi and soil bacteria. Applied Microbiology Biotechnology. 2011;**89**:917-930. doi: 10.1007/s00253-010-3004-6

[54] Nuccio EE, Hodge A, Pett-Ridge J, Herman DJ, Weber PK, Firestone MK. An arbuscular mycorrhizal fungus significantly modifies the soil bacterial community and nitrogen cycling during litter decomposition. Environmental Microbiology. 2013;15:1870-1881. doi: 10.1111/1462-2920.12081

[55] Mankau R. Biological control of nematodes pests by natural enemies. Annual Review of Phytopathology. 1980;**18**:415-440

[56] Jatala P. Biological control of plant-parasitic nematodes. Annual Review of Phytopathology. 1986;**24**:453-489

[57] Tranier M, Pognant-Gros J, De la Cruz Quiroz R, González C, Mateille T, Roussos S. Commercial Biological Control Agents Targeted Against Plant-Parasitic Root-knot Nematodes. Brazilian Archives of Biology and Technology. 2014;**57**:831-841. http://dx.doi.org/10.1590/S1516-8913201402540

[58] Siddiqui ZA, Mahmood I. Role of bacteria in the management of plant-parasitic nematodes: A review. Bioresource Technology. 1999;**69**:167-179

[59] Emmert EAB, Handelsman J. Biocontrol of plant disease: A (Gram) positive perspective. FEMS Microbiology Letters. 1999;**171**:1-9

[60] Meyer SLF. United States Department of Agriculture—Agricultural Research Service research programs on microbes for management of plant-parasitic nematodes. Pest Management Science. 2003;**59**:665-670

[61] Abd-Elgawad MMM, Vagelas IK. Nematophagous Bacteria: Field Application and Commercialization. In: Askary TH, Martinelli PRP, editors. Biocontrol Agents of Phytonematodes. UK: CAB International; 2015. pp. 276-309. 10.1079/9781780643755.0276

[62] Sayre RM, Starr MP. *Pasteuria penetrans* (ex Thorne 1940) non. rev. comb. n. sp. n. a mycelial and endospore forming bacterium parasite in plant parasitic nematodes. Proceedings of the Helminthological Society of Washington. 1985;**52**:149-165

[63] Bekal S, Borneman J, Springer MS, Giblin-Davis RM, Becker JO. Phenotypic and molecular analysis of a *Pasteuria* strain parasitic to the sting nematode. Journal of Nematology. 2001;**33**:110-115

[64] Kun XC, Jun LX, Qin XJ, Lei G, Qun DC, He MM, Qin ZK, Xiang YF, Huang FD. Phylogenetic analysis of the nematicidal actinobacteria from agricultural soil of China. African Journal of Microbiology Research. 2011;**5**(16):2316-2324

[65] Mishra SK, Keller JE, Miller JR, Heisey RM, Nair MG, Putnam AR. Insecticidal and nematicidal properties of microbial metabolites. Indian Journal of Microbiology. 1987;**2**:267-276

[66] Dicklow MB, Acosta N, Zuckerman BM. A novel *Streptomyces* species for controlling plant-parasitic nematodes. Journal of Chemical Ecology. 1993;**19**:159-173

[67] Nour SM, Lawrence JR, Zhu H, Swerhone GDW, Welsh M, Welacky TW, Topp E. Bacteria associated with cysts of the soybean cyst nematode (*Heterodera glycines*). Applied Environmental Microbiology. 2003;**69**:607-615

[68] Burg RW, Miller BM, Baker EE, Birnbaum J, Currie SA, Hartman R, Kong YL, Richard L, Monaghan RL, Olsonm G, Putter I, Tunac JB, Wwllick H, Stapley EO, Oiwa R, Omura S. Avermectins, new family of potent anthelmintic agents: Producing organism and fermentation. Antimicrobial Agents and Chemotherapy. 1979;**15**:361-367

[69] Sun MH, Li G, Shi YX, Li BJ, Liu XZ. Fungi and actinomycetes associated with *Meloidogyne* spp. eggs and females in China and their biocontrol potential. Journal of Invertebrate Pathology. 2006;**93**:22-28

[70] Ruanpanun P, Laatsch H, Tangchitsomkid N, Lumyong S. Nematicidal activity of fervenulin isolated from a nematicidal actinomycete, *Streptomyces* sp. CMU-MH021, on *Meloidogyne incognita.* World Journal of Microbiology and Biotechnology. 2011;**27**(6):1373-1380. doi: 10.1007/s11274-010-0588-z

[71] Kaur T, Jasrotia S, Ohri P, Manhas RK. Evaluation of in vitro and in vivo nematicidal potential of a multifunctional streptomycete, *Streptomyces hydrogenans* strain DH16 against *Meloidogyne incognita*. Microbiological Research. 2016;**192**:247-252. doi: 10.1016/j.micres.2016.07.009

[72] Xiong J. Zhou Q, Luo H, Xia L, Li L, Sun M, Yu Z. Systemic nematicidal activity and biocontrol efficacy of Bacillus firmus against the root-knot nematode *Meloidogyne incognita*. World Journal of Microbiology and Biotechnology. 2015;**31**:661. doi: 10.1007/s11274-015-1820-7

[73] Sayre M, Starr MP. Bacterial diseases and antagonism of nematode. In: Poinar Jr, GO, Jannso HB, editors. Diseases of Nematodes. Boca Raton, FL: CRC Press; 1988. pp. 69-101

[74] Giblin-Davis RM, Williams DS, Bekal S, Dickson DW, Brito JA, Becker JO, Preston JF. *Candidatus Pasteuria* usage sp. nov., an obligate endoparasite of the phytoparasitic nematode *Belonlaimus longicaudatus*. International Journal of Systematic and Evolutionary Microbiology. 2003;**53**:197-200

[75] Mohan S, Mauchline TH, Rowe J, Hirsch PR, Davies KG. *Pasteuria* endospores from *Heterodera cajani* (Nematoda: Heteroderidae) exhibit inverted attachment and altered germination in cross-infection studies with *Globodera pallida* (Nematoda: Heteroderidae). FEMS Microbiology Ecology. 2012;**79**:675-684

[76] Wilson MJ, Jackson TA. Progress in the commercialisation of bionematicides. BioControl. 2013;**58**:715-722

[77] Schüßler AH, Gehrig H, Schwarzott D, Walker C. Analysis of partial Glomales SSU rRNA gene sequences: Implications for primer design and phylogeny. Mycological Research. 2001;**105**:5-15. doi: 10.1017/S0953756200003725

[78] Smith SE, Read DJ. Mineral nutrition, toxic element accumulation and water relations of arbuscular mycorrhizal plants. In: Smith SE, Read DJ, editors. Mycorrhizal Symbiosis. 3rd ed. London: Academic Press; 2008. pp. 145-148

[79] Porcel R, Aroca R, Ruiz-Lozano JM. Salinity stress alleviation using arbuscular mycorrhizal fungi. A review. Agronomy for Sustainable Development. 2011;**32**:181-200. doi: 10.1007/s13593-011-0029-x

[80] Augé RM, Toler HD, Saxton AM. Arbuscular mycorrhizal symbiosis alters stomatal conductance of host plants more under drought than under amply watered conditions: A meta-analysis. Mycorrhiza. 2015;**25**:13-24. doi: 10.1007/s00572-014-0585-4

[81] Tchabi A, Hountondji FCC, Ogunsola B, Lawouin L, Coyne D, Wiemken A, Oehl F. The influence of arbuscular mycorrhizal fungi inoculation on micro-propagated hybrid yam (*Dioscorea* spp.) growth and root-knot nematode (*Meloidogyne* spp.) suppression. International Journal of Current Microbiology and Applied Sciences. 2016;**5**(10):267-281

[82] Ceballos I, Ruiz M, Fernandez C, Pena R, Rodriguez A, Sanders IR. The in vitro mass-produced model mycorrhizal fungus, *Rhizophagus irregularis*, significantly increases yields of the globally important food security crop Cassava. PLoS One. 2013;**8**:e70633. doi: 10.1371/journal.pone.0070633

[83] Khaosaad T, García-Garrido JM, Steinkellner S, Vierheilig H. Take-all disease is systemically reduced in roots of mycorrhizal barley plants. Soil Biology and Biochemistry. 2007;**39**:727-734. 10.1016/j.soilbio.2006.09.014

[84] Castellanos-Morales V, Keiser C, Cárdenas-Navarro R, Grausgruber H, Glauninger J, García-Garrido JM, et al. The bioprotective effect of AM root colonization against the soil-borne fungal pathogen *Gaeumannomyces graminis* var. tritici in barley depends on the barley variety. Soil Biology and Biochemistry. 2011;**43**:831-834. 10.1016/j.soilbio.2010.12.020

[85] Zamioudis C, Pieterse CMJ. Modulation of host immunity by beneficial microbes. Molecular Plant Microbe Interactions. 2012;**25**:139-150. 10.1094/MPMI-06-11-0179

[86] Boller T, Felix G. A renaissance of elicitors: Perception of microbe-associated molecular patterns and danger signals by pattern recognition receptors. Annual Review of Plant Biology. 2009;**60**:379-406

[87] Jones JDG, Dangl JL. The plant immune system. Nature. 2006;**444**:323-329. 10.1038/nature05286

[88] Kloppholz S, Kuhn H, Requena N. A secreted fungal effector of Glomus intraradices promotes symbiotic biotrophy. Current Biology. 2011;**21**:1204-1209

[89] Oldroyd GED, Harrison MJ, Paszkowski U. Reprogramming plant cells for endosymbiosis. Science. 2009;**324**(5928):753-754. doi: 10.1126/science.1171644

[90] Besserer A, Becard G, Jauneau A, Roux C, Sejalon-Delmas N. GR24, a synthetic analog of strigolactones, stimulates the mitosis and growth of the arbuscular mycorrhizal fungus *Gigaspora rosea* by boosting its energy metabolism. Plant Physiology. 2008;**148**:402-413. doi: 10.1104/pp.108.121400

[91] Parniske M. Arbuscular mycorrhiza: The mother of plant root endosymbioses. Nature Reviews Microbiology. 2008;**6**:763-775

[92] Rosas S, Soria R, Correa N, Abdala G. Jasmonic acid stimulates the expression of nod-genes in rhizobium. Plant Molecular Biology. 1998;**38**:1161-1168

[93] Mabood F, Souleimanov A, Khan W, Smith DL. Jasmonates induce Nod factor production by *Bradyrhizobium japonicum*. Plant Physiology and Biochemistry. 2006;**44**:759-765. doi: 10.1038/nrmicro1987

[94] Viaene N, Coyne DL, Kerry BR. Biological and cultural management. In: Perry RN, Moens M, editors. Plant Nematology. Wallingford, UK: CAB International; 2006. pp. 346-369

[95] Yu O, Coosemans J. Fungi associated with cysts of *Globodera rostochiensis, G-pallida,* and *Heterodera schachtii*; and egg masses and females of *Meloidogyne hapla* in Belgium. Phytoprotection. 1998;**79**:63-69. DOI: 10.7202/706135ar

[96] Kerry BR. Rhizosphere interactions and the exploitation of microbial agents for the biological control of plant-parasitic nematodes. Annual Review of Phytopathology. 2000;**38**:423-441. DOI: 10.1146/annurev.phyto.38.1.423

[97] Whitehead AG. Plant Nematode Control. Wallingford, UK: CAB International; 1998. p. 384

[98] Hallmann J, Davies KG, Sikora R. Biological control using microbial pathogens, endophytes and antagonists. In: Perry RN, Moens M, Starr JL, editors. Root-Knot Nematodes. Wallingford, UK: CAB International; 2009. pp. 380-411

[99] Kerry BR, Jaffee BA. Fungi as biological control agents for plant parasitic nematodes. In: Wicklow DT, Soderstrom BE, editors. The Mycota: A Comprehensive Treatise on Fungi as Experimental Systems for Basic and Applied Research, Volume 4 Environmental and Microbial Relationships. Berlin: Springer; 1997. pp. 203-218

[100] Lopez-Llorca LV, Macià-Vicente JG, Jansson H-BJ. Mode of action and interactions of nematophagous fungi. In: Ciancio A, Mukerji KG, editors. Integrated Management and Biocontrol of Vegetable and Grain Crops Nematode. Dordrecht: Springer; 2008. pp. 51-76

[101] Anke H, Stadler M, Mayer A, Sterner O. Secondary metabolites with nematicidal and antimicrobial activity from nematophagous fungi and Ascomycetes. Canadian Journal of Botany. 1995;**73**:932-939. DOI: 10.1139/b95-341

[102] Chet I, Harman GE, Baker R. *Trichoderma hamatum*: Its hyphal interactions with *Rhizoctonia solani* and *Pythium* spp. Microbial Ecology. 1981;**7**:29-38. DOI: 10.1007/BF02010476

[103] Windham GL, Windham MT, Williams WP. Effects of *Trichoderma* spp. on maize growth and *Meloidogyne arenaria* reproduction. Plant Disease. 1989;**73**:493-495. DOI: 10.1094/PD-73-0493

[104] Spiegel Y, Chet I: Evaluation of *Trichoderma* spp. as a biocontrol agent against soilborne fungi and plant-parasitic nematodes in Israel. Integrated Pest Management Review. 1998;**3**:1-7. DOI: 10.1023/A:1009625831128

[105] Sharon E, Chet I, Viterbo A, Bar-Eyal M, Nagan H, Samuels GJ, Spiegel Y. Parasitism of *Trichoderma* on *Meloidogyne javanica* and role of the gelatinous matrix. European Journal of Plant Pathology. 2007;**118**:247-258. DOI: 10.1007/s10658-007-9140-x

[106] Affokpon A, Coyne DL, De Proft M, Coosemans J. In vitro growth characterization and biocontrol potential of naturally occurring nematophagous fungi recovered from

root-knot nematode infested vegetable fields in Benin. International Journal of Pest Management. 2015;**61**:273-283. DOI: 10.1080/09670874.2015.1043971

[107] Chet I, Inbar J, Hadar Y. Fungal antagonists and mycoparasitism. In: Wicklow DT, Soderstrom BE, editors. The Mycota. Volume IV: Environmental and Microbial Relationships. Heidelberg: Springer-Verlag; 1997. pp. 165-184

[108] Howell CR. Mechanisms employed by *Trichoderma* species in the biological control of plant diseases: The history and evolution of current concepts. Plant Disease. 2003;**87**:4-10. DOI: 10.1094/PDIS.2003.87.1.4

[109] Rodríguez-Kábana R, Morgan-Jones G, Godroy G, Gintis BO. Effectiveness of species of *Gliocladium*, *Paecilomyces* and *Verticillium* for control of *Meloidogyne arenaria* in field soil. Nematropica. 1984;**14**:155-170

[110] Freitas LG, Ferraz S, Muchovey JJ. Effectiveness of different isolates of *Paecilomyces lilacinus* and an isolate of *Cylindorcarpon destructans* on the control of *Meloidogyne javanica*. Nematropica. 1995;**25**:109-115

[111] Goswami J, Pandey RK, Tewari JP, Goswami BK. Management of root knot nematode on tomato through application of fungal antagonists, *Acremonium strictum* and *Trichoderma harzianum*. Journal of Environmental Science and Health. 2008;**43**:237-240. DOI: 10.1080/03601230701771164

[112] Sikora RA, Schönbeck F. Effect of vesicular-arbuscular mycorrhizae, *Endogone mosseae* on the population dynamics of the root-knot nematodes *Meloidogyne incognita* and *M. hapla*. In: Proceedings of the 8th International Congress of Plant Protection; 21-27 August 1975; Moscow. pp. 158-166

[113] Jeffries P, Gianinazzi S, Perotto S, Turnau K, Barea JM. The contribution of arbuscular mycorrhizal fungi in sustainable maintenance of plant health and soil fertility. Biology and Fertility of Soils. 2003;**37**:1-16. DOI: 10.1007/s00374-002-0546-5

[114] Harley JL, Smith SE. Mycorrhizal Symbiosis. London: Academic Press; 1983. p. 483

[115] Bonfante-Fasolo P. Anatomy and morphology VA mycorrhizae. In: Powell CL, Bagyaraj DJ, editors. VA Mycorrhiza. Boca Raton: CRC Press; 1984. pp. 5-32

[116] Peyronel B, Fassi B, Fontana A, Trappe JM. Terminology of mycorrhizae. Mycologia. 1969;**61**:410-441

[117] Azcón-Aguilar C, Barea JM. Arbuscular mycorrhizas and biological control of soil-borne plant pathogens—An overview of the mechanisms involved. Mycorrhiza. 1996;**6**:457-464. DOI:10.1007/s005720050147

[118] Ruiz-Lozano JM. Arbuscular mycorrhizal symbiosis and alleviation of osmotic stress: New perspectives for molecular studies. Mycorrhiza. 2003;**13**:309-317. DOI: 10.1007/s00572-003-0237-6

[119] Whipps JM. Prospects and limitations for mycorrhizals in biocontrol of root pathogens. Canadian Journal of Botany. 2004;**82**:1198-1227. DOI: 10.1139/b04-082

[120] Elsen A, Gervacio D, Swennen R, De Waele D. AMF-induced biocontrol against plant parasitic nematodes in *Musa* sp.: A systemic effect. Mycorrhiza. 2008;**18**:251-256. DOI: 10.1007/s00572-008-0173-6

[121] Hallmann J, Sikora RA. Influence of *F. oxysporum*, a mutualistic fungal endophyte on *M. incognita* on tomato. Journal of Plant Diseases and Protection. 1994a;**101**:475-481

[122] Dababat AA, Sikora RA. Induced resistance by the mutualistic endophyte, *Fusarium oxysporum* strain 162, toward *Meloidogyne incognita* on tomato. Biocontrol Science and Technology. 2007a;**17**:969-975. DOI:10.1080/09583150701582057

[123] Dababat AA, Sikora RA. Influence of the mutualistic endophyte *Fusarium oxysporum* 162 on *Meloidogyne incognita* attraction and invasion. Nematology. 2007b;**9**:771-776. DOI: 10.1163/156854107782331225

[124] Kerry BR. Exploitation of the nematophagous fungal *Verticillium chlamydosporium* Goddard for the biological control of root knot nematodes (*Meloidogyne* spp.). In: Butt MT, Jackson CW, Magan N, editors. Fungi as Biocontrol Agents-Progress, Problems and Potential. Wallingford, UK: CAB International; 2001. pp. 155-166

[125] Zare R, Gams W. A revision of *Verticillium* sect. *Prostrata*. III. Generic classification. Nova Hedwigia. 2001;**72**:329-337

[126] Chen S, Dickson DW. Biological control of nematodes by fungal antagonists. In: Chen ZX, Chen SY, Dickson DW, editors. Nematology Advances and Perspectives. Volume II Nematode Management and Utilization. Wallingford, UK: CAB International; 2004. pp. 977-1039

[127] Kerry BR, Bourne JM. The importance of rhizosphere interactions in the biological control of plant parasitic nematodes—a case study using *Verticillium chlamydosporium*. Pesticide Science. 1996;**47**:69-75. DOI: 10.1002/(SICI)1096-9063(199605)47:1<69::AID-PS386>3.0.CO;2-6

[128] Jalali AAH, Segers R, Coosemans J. Biocontrol of *Heterodera schachtii* using combinations of the sterile fungus, StFCh1-1, *Embellisia chlamydospora* and *Verticillium chlamydosporium*. Nematologica. 1998;**44**:345-355. DOI: 10.1163/005525998X00025

[129] Lysek H, Sterba J. Colonization of *Ascaris lumbricoides* eggs by the fungus *Verticillium chlamydosporium* Goddard. Folia Parasitologica. 1991;**8**:255-259

[130] Segers R, Butt TM, Kerry BR, Beckett A, Peberdy JF. The role of the proteinase VCP1 produced by the nematophagous *Verticillium chlamydpsporium* in the infection process of nematode eggs. Mycological Research. 1996;**100**:421-428

[131] Morton CO, Hirsch AM, Kerry BR. Infection of plant-parasitic nematodes by nematophagous fungi—A review of the application of molecular biology to understand infection processes and to improve biological control. Nematology. 2004;**6**:161-170. DOI: 10.1163/1568541041218004

[132] Dackman C. Fungal parasites of the potato cyst nematode *Globodera rostochiensis:* Isolation and reinfection. Journal of Nematology. 1990;**22**:594-597

[133] Kerry BR, De Leij AAM. Key factors in the development of fungal agents for the control of cyst and root-knot nematodes. In: Tjamos EC, Papavizas GC, Cook RJ, editors. Biological Control of Plant Diseases. New York, NY: Plenum Press; 1992. pp. 139-144

[134] De Leij FAAM, Kerry BR. The nematophagous fungus *Verticillium chlamydosporium* Goddard, as a potential biological control agent for *Meloidogyne arenaria* (Neal) Chitwood. Revue de Nématologie. 1991;**14**:157-164

[135] Bourne JM, Kerry BR, De Leij FAAM. The importance of the host plant in the interaction between root-knot nematodes (*Meloidogyne* spp.) and the nematophagous fungus *Verticillium chlamydosporium* Goddard. Biocontrol Science and Technology. 1996;**6**:539-548. DOI: 10.1080/09583159631172

[136] Kerry BR, Bourne JM. A Manual for Research on *Verticillium chlamydosporium*, a Potential Biological Control Agent for Root-Knot Nematodes. Darmstadt: Druckform GmbH; 2002. p. 84

[137] De Oca NM, Arévalos J, Nuñez A, Riverón Y, Villoch A, Hidalgo-Díaz L. KlamiC: Experiencia técnica-productiva. Revista de Protección Vegetal. 2009;**24**:62-65

[138] Esposito E, Da Silva M. Systematics and environmental application of the genus *Trichoderma*. Critical Reviews in Microbiology. 1998;**24**:89-98. DOI: 10.1080/10408419891294190

[139] Harman GE, Howell CR, Viterbo A, Chet I, Lorito M. *Trichoderma* species—Opportunistic, avirulent plant symbionts. Nature Reviews, Microbiology. 2004;**2**:43-56. DOI: 10.1038/nrmicro797

[140] Kyalo G, Affokpon A, Coosemans J, Coyne DL. Biological control effects of *Pochonia chlamydosporia* and *Trichoderma* isolates from Benin (West-Africa) on root-knot nematodes. Communications in Agricultural and Applied Biological Sciences. 2007;**72**:219-223

[141] Affokpon A, Coyne DL, Htay CC, Dossou Agbèdè R, Lawouin L, Coosemans J. Biocontrol potential of native *Trichoderma* isolates against root-knot nematodes in West African vegetable production systems. Soil Biology and Biochemistry. 2011a;**43**:600-608. DOI: 10.1016/j.soilbio.2010.11.029

[142] Kullnig-Gradinger CM, Szakacs G, Kubicek CP. Phylogeny and evolution of the fungal genus *Trichoderma*-a multigene approach. Mycological Research. 2002;**106:**757-767. DOI: 10.1017/S0953756202006172

[143] Yedidia I, Benhamou N, Chet I. Induction of defense response in cucumber plants (*Cucumis sativus* L.) by the biocontrol agent *Trichoderma harzianum*. Applied Environmental Microbiology. 1999;**65**:1061-1070

[144] Sikora RA, Oka Y, Sharon, E, Hok CJ, Keren-Zur M. Achievements and research requirements for the integration of biocontrol into farming systems. Nematology. 2000;**2**:737-738. DOI: 10.1163/156854100509592

[145] Bennett AJ, Mead A, Whipps JM. Performance of carrot and onion seed primed with beneficial microorganisms in glasshouse and field trials. Biological Control. 2009;**51**:417-426. DOI: 10.1016/j.biocontrol.2009.08.001

[146] Rilling MC, Wright SF, Eviner VT. The role of arbuscular mycorrhizal fungi and glomalin in soil aggregation: Comparing effects of five plant species. Plant and Soil. 2002;**238**:325-333. DOI: 10.1023/A:1014483303813

[147] Tchabi A, Burger S, Coyne D, Hountondji F, Lawouin L, Wiemken A, Oehl F. Promiscuous arbuscular mycorrhizal symbiosis of yam (*Dioscorea* spp.), a key staple crop in West Africa. Mycorrhiza. 2009;**19**:375-392. DOI: 10.1007/s00572-009-0241-6

[148] Tchabi A, Coyne D, Hountondji F, Lawouin L, Wiemken A, Oehl F. Efficacy of indigenous arbuscular mycorrhizal fungi for promoting white yam (*Dioscorea rotundata*) growth in West Africa. Applied Soil Ecology. 2010;**45**:92-100. DOI: 10.1016/j.apsoil.2010.03.001

[149] Davies JFT, Puryear JD, Newton RJ, Egilla JN, Saraiva Grossi SJA. Mycorrhizal fungi enhance accumulation and tolerance of chromium in sunflower (*Helianthus annuus*). Journal of Plant Physiology. 2001;**158**:777-786. DOI: 10.1078/0176-1617-00311

[150] Chen BD, Roos P, Borggaard OK, Zhu Y-G, Jakobsen I. Mycorrhiza and root hairs in barley enhance acquisition of phosphorus and uranium from phosphate rock but mycorrhiza decreases root to shoot uranium transfer. *New Phytologists*. 2005;**165**:591-598. DOI: 10.1111/j.1469-8137.2004.01244.x

[151] Al-Karaki GN. Benefit, cost and water-use efficiency of arbuscular mycorrhizal during wheat grown under drought stress. Mycorrhiza. 1998;**8**:41-45. DOI: 10.1007/s005720050209

[152] Jaizme-Vega MC, Tenoury P, Pinochet J, Jaumot M. Interactions between the root-knot nematode *Meloidogyne incognita* and *Glomus mosseae* in banana. Plant and Soil. 1997;**196**:27-35. DOI:10.1023/A:1004236310644

[153] Declerck, S, Risèd JM, Rufyikiri G, Delvaux B. Effects of arbuscular mychorrhizal fungi on severity of root rot of bananas caused by *Cylindrocladium spathiphylli*. Plant Pathology. 2002;**51**:109-115. DOI: 10.1046/j.0032-0862.2001.656.x

[154] Gange AC, Brown VK, Aplin D. Multitrophic links between arbuscular mycorrhizal fungi and insect parasitoids. Ecology Letters. 2003;**6**:1051-1055. DOI: 10.1046/j.1461-0248.2003.00540.x

[155] Marro N, Lax P, CabelloM, Doucet ME, Becerra AG. Use of the arbuscular mycorrhizal fungus *Glomus intraradices* as biological control agent of the nematode *Nacobbus aberrans* Parasitizing Tomato. Brazilian Archives of Biology and Technology. 2014;**57**:668-674. DOI: 10.1590/S1516-8913201402200.

[156] Mohanty KC, Sahoo NK. Prospects of mycorrhizae as potential nematode antagonist. In: Trivedi PC, editor. Advances in Nematology. India: Scientific Publishers; 2003. p. 317

[157] Hol WHG, Cook R. An overview of arbuscular mycorrhizal fungi-nematode interactions. Basic and Applied Ecology. 2005;**6**:489-503. DOI: 10.1016/j.baae.2005.04.001

[158] Castillo P, Nico AI, Azcón-Aguilar C, Del Río Rincón C, Calvet C, Jiménez-Díaz RM. Protection of olive planting stocks against parasitism of root-knot nematodes by arbuscular mycorrhizal fungi. Plant Pathology. 2006;**55**:705-713. DOI: 10.1111/j.1365-3059.2006.01400.x

[159] Masadeh B, Von Alten H, Grunewaldt-Stoecker G, Sikora RA. Biocontrol of root-knot nematodes using the arbuscular mycorrhizal fungus *Glomus intraradices* and the antagonist *Trichoderma viride* in two tomato cultivars differing in their suitability as hosts for the nematodes. Journal Plant Disease and Protection. 2004;**111**:322-333

[160] Ryan NA, Deliopoulos T, Jones P, Haydock PPJ. Effects of a mixed-isolate mycorrhizal inoculum on the potato-potato cyst nematode interaction. Annals of Applied Biology 2003;**143**:111-119. DOI: 10.1111/j.1744-7348.2003.tb00275.x

[161] Schwob I, Ducher M, Coudret A. Effects of climatic factors on native arbuscular mycorrhizae and *Meloidogyne exigua* in a Brazilian rubber tree (*Hevea brasiliensis*) plantation. Plant Pathology. 1999;**48**:19-25. DOI: 10.1046/j.1365-3059.1999.00300.x

[162] Waceke JW, Waudo SW, Sikora R. Effect of inorganic phosphatic fertilizers on the efficacy of an arbuscular mycorrhiza fungus against a root-knot nematode on pyrethrum. International Journal of Pest Management. 2002;**48**:307-313. DOI: 10.1080/09670870210149862

[163] De La Peña E, Echeverría SR, Van Der Putten HH, Freitas H, Moens M. Mechanism of control of root-feeding nematodes by mycorrhizal fungi in the dune grass *Ammophila arenaria*. New Phytologists. 2006;**169**:829-840. DOI: 10.1111/j.1469-8137.2005.01602.x

[164] Zhang L, Zhang J, Christie P, Li X. Pre-inoculation with arbuscular mycorrhizal fungi suppresses root knot nematode (*Meloidogyne incognita*) on cucumber (*Cucumis sativus*). Biology and Fertility of Soils. 2008;**45**:205-212. DOI: 10.1007/s00374-008-0329-8

[165] Affokpon A, Coyne DL, Lawouin L, Tossou C, Dossou Agbèdè R, Coosemans J. Effectiveness of native West African arbuscular mycorrhizal fungi in protecting vegetable crops against root-knot nematodes. Biology and Fertility of Soils. 2011b;**47**:207-217. DOI 10.1007/s00374-010-0525-1

[166] Diedhiou PM, Hallmann J, Oerke EC, Dehne HW. Effects of arbuscular mycorrhizal fungi and a non-pathogenic *Fusarium oxysporum* on *Meloidogyne incognita* infestation of tomato. Mycorrhiza. 2003;**13**:199-204. DOI 10.1007/s00572-002-0215-4

[167] Rumbos C, Reimann S, Kiewnick S, Sikora RA. Interactions of *Paecilomyces lilacinus* strain 251 with the mycorrhizal fungus *Glomus intraradices*: Implications for *Meloidogyne incognita* control on tomato. Biocontrol Science and Technology. 2006;**16**:981-986. DOI: 10.1080/09583150600937667

[168] Domsch KH, Gams W, Anderson T-H. Compendium of Soil Fungi. London: Academic Press; 1980. p. 406

[169] Jatala P, Kaltenback R, Bocangel M. Biological control of *Meloidogyne acrita* and *Globodera pallida* on potatoes. Journal of Nematology. 1979;**11**:303

[170] Holland RJ, Williams KL, Khan A. Infection of *Meloidogyne javanica* by *Paecilomyces lilacinus*. Nematology. 1999;**1**:131-139. DOI: 10.1163/156854199508090

[171] Kiewnick S, Sikora RA. Biological control of the root-knot nematode *Meloidogyne incognita* by *Paecilomyces lilacinus* strain 251. Biological Control. 2006;**38**:179-187. DOI: 10.1016/j.biocontrol.2005.12.006

[172] Speijer PR. Interrelationships between *Pratylenchus goodeyi* Sher & Allen and strains of nonpathogenic *Fusarium oxysporum* Schl. emd. Snyd. & Hans. in roots of two banana cultivars [thesis]. Bonn: University of Bonn; 1993

[173] Schuster RP, Sikora RA, Amin N. Potential of endophytic fungi for the biological control of plantlet parasitic nematodes. Mededelingen van de Faculteit Landbouwwetenschappen Rijksuniversiteit Gent. 1995;**60**:1047-1052

[174] Griesbach M. Occurrence of mutualistic fungal endophytes in bananas (*Musa* spp.) and their potential as biocontrol agents of banana weevil *Cosmopolites sordidus* (Germar) in Uganda [thesis]. Bonn: University of Bonn; 2000

[175] Hallmann J, Sikora RA. Occurrence of plant parasitic nematodes and nonpathogenic species of Fusarium in tomato plants in Kenya and their role as mutualistic synergists for biological control of root knot nematodes. International Journal of Pest Management. 1994b;**40**:321-325. DOI: 10.1080/09670879409371907

[176] Pocasangre LE. Biological enhancement of banana tissue culture plantlets with endophytic fungi for the control of the burrowing nematode *Radopholus similis* and the Panama disease (*Fusarium oxysporum* f.sp. cubense) [thesis]. Bonn: University of Bonn; 2000

[177] Niere B. Significance of non-pathogenic isolates of *Fusarium oxysporum* Schlecht.: Fries for the biological control of the burrowing nematode *Radopholus similis* (Cobb) Thorne on tissue cultured banana [thesis]. Bonn: University of Bonn; 2001

[178] Vu TT, Hauschild R, Sikora RA. *Fusarium oxysporum* endophytes induced systemic resistance against *Radopholus similis* on banana. Nematology. 2006;**8**:847-852. DOI: 10.1163/156854106779799259

[179] Mennan S, Aksoy HM, Ecevit O. Antagonistic effect of *Fusarium oxysporum* on *Heterodera cruciferae*. Journal of Phytopathology. 2005;**153**:221-225. DOI: 10.1111/j.1439-0434.2005.00957.x.

[180] Waweru BW, Turoop L, Kahangi E, Coyne D, Dubois T. Non-pathogenic Fusarium oxysporum endophytes provide field control of nematodes, improving yield of banana (Musa sp.). Biological Control. 2014;**74**:82-88. DOI: 10.1016/j.biocontrol.2014.04.002

[181] Al kader MAA. In vitro studies on nematode interactions with their antagonistic fungi in the rhizosphere of various plants [thesis]. Freiburg im Breisgau: Universität Freiburg im Breisgau; 2008

[182] Zopf W. Zur kenntnis der infektions-krankheiten niederer thiere und pflanzen. Nova Acta Academiae Caesareae Leopoldino-Carolinae Germanicae Naturae Curiosorum. 1888;**52**:314-376

[183] Niu X-M, Zhang K-Q. *Arthrobotrys oligospora*: A model organism for understanding the interaction between fungi and nematodes. Mycology. 2011;**2**:59-78. DOI: 10.1080/21501203.2011.562559

[184] Saikawa M, Takahashi A. Nonconstricting-ring formation in two species of nematode-capturing hyphomycetes. Mycoscience. 2002;**43**:417-419. DOI: 10.1007/s102670200061

[185] Ferris H, Castro CE, Caswell EP, Jaffee BA, Roberts PA, Westerdahl BB, Williamson VM. Biological approaches to the management of plant-parasitic nematodes. In: Madden JP, editor. Beyond Pesticides: Biological Approaches to Pest Management in California. CA: University of California; 1992. pp. 68-101

[186] Nordbring-Hertz B, Jansson H-B, Tunlid A. Nematophagous fungi. Encyclopedia of Life Science. 2002;**12**:681-690. DOI: 10.1038/npg.els.0004293

[187] Santos MA, Ferraz S, Muchovej JJ. Evaluation of 20 species of fungi from Brazil for biocontrol of *Meloidogyne incognita* race 3. Nematropica. 1992;**22**:183-192

[188] Nordbring-Hertz B, Jansson H-B, Friman E, Persson Y, Dackman C, Hard T, Poloczek E, Feldmann R. Nematophagous Fungi. Film no. V, 1851. Göttingen: Institut für den Wissenschaftlichen Film; 1995

[189] Martin SB. Nematode control. Available at: http://media.clemson.edu/public/turfgrass/2013%20 Pest%20Management/2013_nematode_cont.pdf (accessed 05 may, 2017).

[190] Wang B, Liu XZ. Mass production and formulation of nematode-antagonistic microbes. In: Liu XZ, Zhang KQ, Li TF, editors. Biological Control of Plant-Parasitic Nematodes (in Chinese, with English abstract). Beijing, China: China Science and Technology Press; 2004, pp. 285-297.

[191] Meyer SLF, Roberts· DP, Chitwood DJ, Carta LK, Lumsden RD, Mao W. Application of *Burkholderia cepacia* and *Trichoderma virens*, alone and in combinations, against *Meloidogyne incognita* on bell pepper. Nematropica. 2001;31:75-86.

[192] Raddy HM, Fouad AFA, Montasser SA, Abdel-Lateef MF, El-Samadisy AM. Efficacy of six nematicides and six commercial bioproducts against root-knot nematode, *Meloidogyne incognita* on tomato. Journal of Applied Sciences Research. 2013;9:4410-4417.

[193] Abd-Elgawad MMM, Aboul-Eid HZ. Effects of oxamyl, insect nematodes and *Serratia marcescens* on a polyspecific nematode community and yield of tomato. Egyptian Journal of Agronematology. 2001;5:79-89.

[194] Wei LH, Xue QY, Wei BQ, Wang YM, Li SM, Chen LF, Guo JH. Screening of antagonisticbacterial strains against *Meloidogyne incognita* using protease activity. Biocontrol Science and Technology. 2010;20:739-750.

[195] Abd-Elgawad MMM, Mohamed MMM, El-Gamal NGS. Development of safe chemicaland biological formulations for control of nematodes in cucumber. Egyptian Pharmaceutical Journal. 2008;7:41-50.